Metabolic Health Roadmap

Step-by-Step Epigenetic Guide to Revitalize
Energy Levels, Sharpen Cognitive Function,
Cultivate Emotional Wellbeing and Customize
Nutritional Intake

Brenda Wollenberg

To my incredible family: Mark, our five kids, their partners,
and the growing gaggle of grandkids,
who have been my wellness "science experiment" for the past 40 years
and have not only lived to tell about it
but have thrived—body, mind, and spirit—thank you!

Contents

Introduction

About Brenda

As a recently minted senior ("Oh my goodness, I can't believe I just said that!"), I wake up loving how I look and feel pretty much every morning.

I am rested—with energy to spare—and one of the first things that springs to mind is gratitude for a myriad of people, scenarios, and belongings. I'm clear-headed, optimistic, joyous, fit and strong. I have a deep connection to myself, others, and my understanding of the divine.

When I Look in the Mirror, I Almost Always Like What I See!

I have laugh lines showing how much I've loved my life. I have crow's feet that give evidence of the pain and challenges I have faced. I have abdominal wrinkles that testify to carrying and nurturing five exceptional, now-adult children.

And, I have surprisingly cool-looking grey hair that showed up super early (as with my dad and grandfather), which is not only genetic but proof of the 40+ years spent with my partner working on creating the best marriage and family life possible.

And amidst all that, I hope and believe that the best years of my life are still ahead of me.

I Didn't, However, Always Look and Feel this Way

Decades ago, long before the human genome had been mapped and "epigenetics" became a more familiar term, I was a sick and often anxious social worker who'd come to that existence on the tail end of a sickly and often anxiety-ridden childhood.

I was tired (as in all the time), carrying excess body fat, stressed and anxious, dealing with insomnia and hypothyroidism, and, truthfully, was pessimistic pretty much every day.

I had rheumatic fever at five years of age and was put on a small dose of daily antibiotics for the next seven years. I had approximately four major colds a year. Each lasting what felt like a season in duration!

While I have good memories of my upbringing, they are woven through with threads of ongoing mental and emotional ache fostered by challenging family of origin events. Thankfully, my physical heart stayed healthy, but my immune system, mental well-being, digestive health, and emotional heart all took a huge hit.

My journey from illness to body|mind|spirit wellness took several years, with numerous missteps and detours along the way. I worked with a number of health practitioners to shift my dietary intake, my exercise patterns, my sleep, and the way I self-regulated. To this day, I am incredibly grateful for the journey and would not be where I am without the discoveries and tools I've learned along the way.

In the 20/20 vision that hindsight often offers, I now see that I "accidentally" reset my genes by utilizing the hallmarks of the concept of epigenetics, a term first introduced by the British embryologist Conrad Waddington in 1942.

Waddington coined the term to describe the complex interactions between genes (the DNA material inherited from our biological parents) and their environment (the things we do to ourselves—diet, stress management, movement—and that happen around us).

Though the term "epigenetics" is tossed around relatively lightly today, this concept was revolutionary then. For the first time, it was recognized that while the genetic code itself couldn't be altered, environmental factors could influence gene expression.

Waddington's early work laid some excellent foundations for a better understanding of how what we do impacts how our genes behave.

I'm not going to lie, however; I would have loved it if he or some other knowledgeable scientist or health practitioner had offered me a simple, sensible, and sustainable shortcut (epigenetic hacks, as it were) to optimal health! Thus, *Metabolic Health Roadmap.*

If you are also looking for a better way to better wellness, you're in the right place.

Prologue

The Starting Line

Pre-Trip Preparation

O K. Let's begin to discover a series of epigenetic steps as your best method to foster increased metabolic health and wellness.

First, a couple of clarifying points, starting with some science.

Epigenetics in Everyday Language

The word "epigenetics" comes from the Greek "epi," which means over or above, so over or above the genome, our actual DNA material. It is a relatively new scientific discipline—the human genome has, after all, only been mapped for a little over 20 years, and Waddington only coined the term six decades before that monumental mapping, which involves studying how the environment changes gene expression. DNA doesn't change. Genes don't change. However, a gene's expression can be altered through environmental cues.

In short, epigenetics relates to factors "on top of" or "in addition to" innate genetic makeup, wellness factors like diet, sleep, exercise and stress management.

Our growing awareness that, for the most part, nurture trumps nature has led to a deeper understanding of the meaning of "environment" and how it impacts gene expression. Everything we do in our daily routines—diet, sleep, movement, calming—supports our DNA's genetic expression for the good or the challenging. That means that lifestyle choices have the potential to go a long way toward increasing energy, strengthening focus, balancing moods and having your body maintain a comfortable-for-you size.

Cell Biology 101

Let's start with a short lesson on DNA (which, if you don't completely understand, will make no difference in the positive changes this book's recommendations can make in your metabolic health and epigenetic outcomes!).

DNA is a long chain of molecules in each cell, passed down from your biological parents. It provides all the information needed for cells to differentiate, reproduce and grow.

Each strand of DNA you inherit—one from each of your parents—comprises many genes, the basic units of heredity. A gene is the portion of that DNA that codes for a specific molecule, usually a particular protein. When you look at the exact code in your genes, you can see whether it is more or less likely they produce a functional protein to make the essential building blocks to create healthy cells.

DNA coding is made up of nitrogenous bases or "letters," Adenine (A), Guanine (G), Cytosine (C) and Thymine (T), that a cell then "reads" as instructions. An allele is a variation of these "letters." If the gene contains a Single Nucleotide Polymorphism (SNP), a variation on the normal code, the SNP may disrupt the gene's message or protein translation; think "typo."

Single nucleotide polymorphisms occur normally in a person's DNA. Each SNP represents a genetic variation within a single DNA building block in a gene sequence called a nucleotide.

While variants are sometimes beneficial, in general, if you have a SNP variant, the protein that the gene produces may not be supportive of cell health.

Many SNPs do not affect health, but some can impact wellness outcomes. "Normal" or ancestral alleles are usually the most common and generally have the least risk of fostering health challenges. "Risk" or variant alleles are generally the least common and are most likely to promote increased health challenges. And there are always exceptions to these "rules" which may make things more complex.

So what does that mean for everyday life?

In simple terms (and ones that would likely have my biologist business partner—with a PhD in Botany —rolling her eyes!), think of the genes you were given at conception as the switches on an electrical panel, like in your basement, laundry room or garage. Each gene "switch" is either flipped one way (homozygous for normal—you got the normal version of the gene from both of your folks) or flipped the other way (homozygous for variant—you got the variant version of the gene from both of your folks). Or, you got a normal version from one parent and a variant version from the other and are heterozygous for that gene. Your gene "electrical panel switch" for a heterozygous coding would be midway between fully on and entirely off.

Now, imagine that a power surge hits the panel. Power surges run the gambit from adverse childhood events to sound nutrition, being in a car accident, practicing an effective self-regulation tool, having a baby, starting a new job, and caring for an aging parent. Those surges impact gene expression. The inflammation from whiplash, for example, can negatively affect up to 90% of your genes. A surge of stress hormones like cortisol, epinephrine and norepinephrine can do likewise.

Implemented and regularly acted upon, however, a series of wellness practices that have you eat optimally for your body type, foster sound sleep, encourage movement that brings you joy and help with stress management can produce a surge of another kind. A surge that optimizes positive gene expression enhances metabolic health and produces energy, clarity and balance.

Genes carry information. "Surges" influence whether or not a gene releases the correct information.

Putting into practice more of the behaviours that have been shown to impact gene expression positively is, in a nutshell, an epigenetic hack. While I won't hit you over the head with that specific phrase much in the following pages, know that each wellness action that resonates with you and you follow through on is an epigenetic hack ... a behaviour that positively impacts gene expression!

Do I Need to Have My DNA Tested to Benefit from Epigenetic Work?

In a word, no. Many of my clients have yet to have their DNA tested. We follow the best practices and principles outlined in this book.

For clients with DNA testing, we work very specifically on a wellness protocol that optimizes their gene expression. We can determine their ideal daily protein, saturated fat, and carbohydrate intake. We can precisely identify whether their body responds best to endurance exercise or High-Intensity Interval Training and develop best-practice self-regulation tools for their short and long-term stress response genes.

Regardless of their genetics, however, I have them set those specifics based on practices that improve metabolic health. The No Matter Whats (NMWs) I speak about in this book are the same NMWs my clients get. We will tweak those basics per raw genetic data, but everyone starts with the principles described here.

Moving on to the next bit of science, metabolic health, I'll start with the news this is a quick-fix diet book. If you're looking for a one-size-fits-all magic bullet, you'll not find it here (or, truth be told, anywhere!).

Instead, metabolic health looks at the processes involved in the body's normal functioning (as our genes dictate). It covers ways to support your many physiological systems to best foster a healthy metabolic state sensibly and sustainably (you'll hear me mention that often!).

Why is metabolic health important?

Put simply, these are the systems within the body that maintain life, including how cells use the fuel we provide—our daily food intake. These processes include breaking down nutrients from our diet to produce energy, synthesizing necessary compounds, building new molecules, and eliminating waste products.

What Does Metabolic Health Look Like?

Recall how I just described how I look and feel each morning. That.

In a slightly more science-informed description, metabolic health can be defined as a state where all the metabolic processes in the body function optimally.

It is characterized by adequate energy production and utilization ("get up and go"); balanced hormone levels (everything from libido to sense of joy and motivation to ability to deeply feel emotions such as grief and loss); effective processing of toxins and aged cellular material (reusing of raw materials and waste disposal); and the body's ability to maintain homeostasis (keeping body systems in a state of balance).

If you want a straight-up clinical definition, you would examine markers such as blood glucose, triglycerides, low-density lipoprotein (LDL) cholesterol, high-density lipoprotein (HDL) cholesterol, blood pressure, and waist circumference. Bearing in mind that these tests typically only give "snapshot" measurements of how one is doing at the time of testing, metabolically healthy people typically have optimal levels of those critical factors.

This, in turn, will reduce the risk of developing the types of diseases that poor metabolic health can contribute to, such as metabolic syndrome, diabetes, cardiovascular disease, and other related conditions.

How Does Metabolic Typing Fit into Metabolic Health?

Metabolic or body typing is a concept we'll cover more thoroughly in Leg 3. Its premise is that personalized wellness is the route to optimal health, based on the idea that each of us has unique metabolic needs.

A primary principle underlying metabolic typing is that people metabolize nutrients differently based on their genetic makeup (those "normal" and "variant" codings, again). As a result of that bio-individuality, different diets and lifestyle choices are better suited for different individuals.

Metabolic Typing Classification

Metabolic typing categorizes people according to one of three metabolic types. In this book, we'll call those three categories:

- **Protein Type:** These individuals typically thrive on higher-protein, higher-fat diets with lower carbohydrate intake. They are often characterized as fast oxidizers, meaning they burn carbohydrates quickly and thus require more protein and fat to sustain energy.

- **Carbohydrate Type:** These individuals typically require higher carbohydrate intake with lower protein and fat intake. They are usually slow oxidizers with a slower rate of carbohydrate metabolism and, in comparison to Protein Types, have more sustained energy with carbohydrate intake.

- **Balanced Type:** Balanced or Mixed types have a relatively balanced oxidation rate and require a more uniform ratio of proteins, fats, and carbohydrates in their food intake.

Benefits of Knowing Your Metabolic Type

Understanding your metabolic type can significantly enhance your metabolic health in several ways:

1. **Optimized Fuel Mix:** Customizing your food intake per your metabolic type can lead to increased energy, improved gut health, and easier maintenance of a comfortable-for-you body size. For example, if you're a Protein Type, increasing your intake of proteins and fats while reducing carbohydrates could lead to stabilized blood sugar and energy levels.

2. **Improved Nutrient Absorption:** Eating in line with your metabolic type can enhance your absorption and utilization of nutrients, reducing the likelihood of nutritional deficiencies and improving overall wellness.

3. **Enhanced Mood and Energy Levels:** Many clients find that eating according to their metabolic type helps stabilize mood fluctuation and

increase energy levels. Again, it is likely that more stable blood sugar levels and better nutrient absorption play a role.

4. **Reduced Incidence of Metabolic Disorders:** Tailoring your diet to your unique metabolic needs can help prevent common disorders such as insulin resistance, diabetes, and obesity, often exacerbated by dietary intake not in line with an individual's unique metabolic needs.

5. **Customized Health Management:** Knowing your metabolic type can also help one fine-tune other aspects of wellness, including the type of movement that might prove most beneficial, the ideal amount and timing of sleep, and optimal stress management tools.

Metabolic typing helps individuals customize their health journey. When you factor genetic predisposition and current health status into your wellness plans, you are more likely to achieve better overall metabolic health and well-being. An individualized approach focuses on the preventative aspect of the illness/wellness equation and on fostering a higher quality of life overall.

What You'll Find Here

Metabolic Health Roadmap is an essential guide to using epigenetic hacks to produce optimal wellness.

It gives simple steps for:

- Eating soundly for your metabolic type.

- Moving in ways that bring vitality.

- Engaging in the types of rest that will most restore you.

- Dealing with stress in ways that are manageable and life-giving.

Want more out of life—physically, mentally and emotionally? Are you prepared to learn (and unlearn) concepts that will help move you forward on the optimal health journey? Ready for a game plan you'll use for life? Then you're in the right place!

Metabolic Health Roadmap - Your Interactive Guide

When embarking on a journey, wellness or otherwise, it's crucial to know where you're going and how you'll get there.

The first Leg of your trip—Prep for Metabolic Health—is where you'll discover what each step entails, see a clear outline of how to use this book (including a handy-dandy two-page Roadmap to Wellness!), and understand why completing your complimentary *Trip Log* brings increased wellness bonuses for you.

"What's that," you say, "A free *Trip Log*?"

It's your tool for tracking what you learn on your journey and listing the tools you decide to implement to best stay on track. It's a brilliant and time-tested manner of reaching your destination.

While you can do any "homework" or journaling in a digital file or paper journal, I've created a *Trip Log* to make "keeping track" simple and coordinated with the trip Legs. This is where you'll take notes, do RoadWork, and create the foundation for your Gutsy Recovery Of Wellness Plan (more on that GROW Plan in Leg 6!).

You can click here to download your free copy of the *Trip Log*. (https://www.inbalancelm.com/MHR_triplog).

Next Up ... Reader Type

(Did you even know you had one???)

Over many years of working with many people, I've realized there are three types of readers: skimmers, deep divers and pickers & choosers. I'm a deep diver. A lover of research. A tell-me-more reader.

WHAT'S YOUR "READER" TYPE?

DEEP-DIVERS	SKIMMERS	PICKERS & CHOOSERS
Oh, tell me more!	**Just the facts, please!**	**I like a little of both!**
These are the wellness content hungry, research-junkies who love to understand all the reasons why their energy is low, and everything they need to do to improve it. This entire book is for you; take it all in!	Folks who want their map for the optimal health journey to be "short and sweet" land here. They want more energy so will seriously consider the suggestions, but want them in bullet point form please!	Have differing "reader" types depending on the circumstances? If time and interest dictate picking and choosing, check the graphics and summaries first and then go for a deeper dive when you choose.

What's Your Reader Type?

That means whatever I write tends to have a lot of content—a "don't-get-me-started, or I'll talk your ear off" amount of content. I want you to understand why I suggest a wellness tool or practice, how it works, the results, and the easiest way to get those results.

Bottom line? Skimmers generally love my practical, doable information but are not keen on how it's delivered. They want beneficial wellness information but sometimes find it a pain in their seating area to extract just the nuts and bolts.

So, thanks to my good friend, fellow nutritionist—and the scientist business partner I mentioned—Alicia, a die-hard skimmer (and someone who has, for ten years, been telling me to "say it shorter"), this book is written with every reader type in mind!

Do you love understanding all the "whys" and hearing stories about what happens when people follow through with *Metabolic Health Roadmap* guidelines? Have at 'er. Deep dive until you have to fight to the surface for sweet, non-word-filled air!

Do you want it short and sweet?

Head for anything graphic or condensed, including each section's summary, the Travel Size Version. The illustrations might not be worth 1000 words, but they'll come close. And the Travel Size Version—the first page of each Leg of the *Metabolic Health Roadmap*—gives you just the basics. If you're intrigued enough to dig further, keep reading the rest of the section.

Yes, that's right; I care so much about supporting skimmers that the summaries are at the start of each Leg (thanks, again, to Alicia).

And for those of you who like to Pick & Choose, you can . . . pick and choose!

Skim for starters and deep dive when you have more time or where your attention is drawn.

And because I don't diagnose or treat in my scope of practice as a nutritionist, please read the medical disclaimer that follows. It's important!

Medical Disclaimer:

There is one last essential point before we start Leg 1, which will pertain to every Leg of the journey. Nutritionists do not diagnose or treat disease. Any information I discuss is meant to supplement the medical counsel of your physician. It's always a good idea to talk with your doctor or healthcare practitioner before making dietary, exercise or other wellness changes, especially if you are pregnant, nursing or have health challenges.

Chapter One

LEG 1 – Prep for Metabolic Health

SUMMARY – Travel Size Version

Where, in This Leg, You'll Get a Lay of the Land

What's a Leg, And What Pre-Trip Prep Do I Need to Know?

Think of a "Leg" as a section in your journey toward enhanced health, with each of the six sets of chapters in this book representing one Leg.

Looking for additional pre-trip tips? Don't miss the helpful graphic that follows on the next page where you'll discover simple tips to:

- Turn Off

- Take Notes

- Top Up

- Tune In

STARTING THE JOURNEY

1	2	3	4
Turn Off	**Take Notes**	**Top Up**	**Tune In**
Anything that might be distracting: phone, computer, music, TV or other devices.	Use your *Trip Log* to journal, do the *Road Work* and see which options resonate with YOU.	You can't think well if you're hungry or thirsty. Plug in the kettle or fuel as needed!	A "Just the facts Ma'am" or deep dive reader; do metabolic health your way!

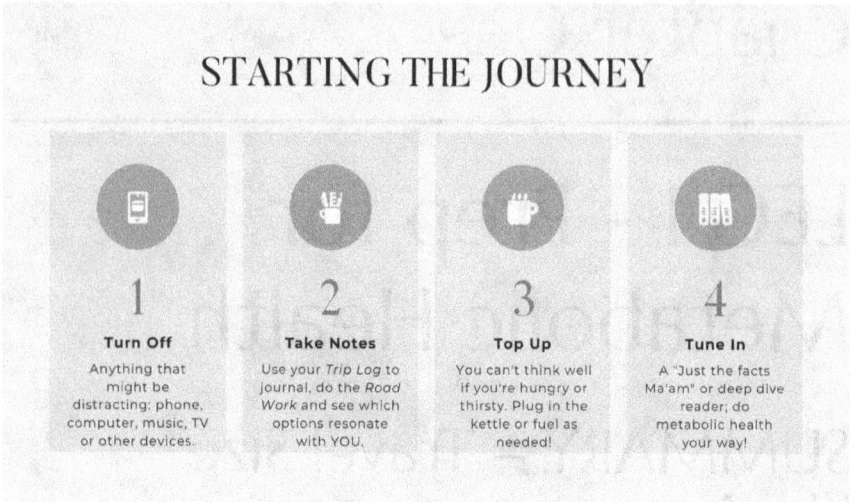

Starting the Metabolic Health Journey

What Exactly Do You Do in a Leg?

In each Leg, you'll . . .

Visit the Information Centre:

Gauge where you're starting with diagnostics—check your oil, assess your tire pressure, and evaluate your gas tank's fullness, as it were. You'll set your wellness destination goals here, absorb new knowledge, and conduct assessments.

Take a Rest Stop:

Pause to digest this information. Spend 10 minutes in calm reflection on the questions provided, then another 10 minutes in quiet, allowing thoughts to pass through your mind like birds—observe them without letting them nest.

Healthy living isn't just about absorbing information—it's about integration. Regular Rest Stops allow you to reflect on and respond to what you've learned, ensuring the journey is as impactful as possible.

Do Some RoadWork:

Engage in one small, impactful activity chosen from two options.

The suggested activities in RoadWork are tried and true, honed through extensive real-life application, and simple yet transformative. Taken in tandem with other Metabolic Health practices, they are designed to integrate smoothly into your daily routine and can revolutionize how you look and feel.

Track Your Progress in a *Trip Log:*

Documenting your journey is crucial. Use pen and paper, digital notes, or the *Trip Log,* which you can download here (https://www.inbalancelm.com/MHR_triplog) to note significant "aha" moments, answer Rest Stop questions, and plan your RoadWork activities. This record will be your roadmap, helping you navigate from where you are to where you want to be.

Receive Traveller Assistance:

Discover body|mind|spirit tools that support your journey. These tools are relevant not just for a specific Leg but as enduring strategies for wellness.

Each tool provided is adaptable, much like a multi-bit screwdriver, perfect for tweaking to fit your unique wellness blueprint.

Pick Up A Souvenir:

Each Leg offers at least one souvenir suggestion, a token of achievement to motivate and mark your progress. These are your celebrations of each milestone reached.

Road Blocks and Traffic Jams

Two primary thought patterns contribute to an inability to move forward wellness-wise.

Unsound Information - Roadblocks (think detour signs): You may encounter detours like misguided beliefs fueled by the food industry's misleading interests or the notion that more effort equals better health.

Unsound Thinking - Traffic Jams (think rush hour traffic): Tackle bottle-necks like misinterpreting the reasons behind your actions, which can lead to self-condemnation instead of self-compassion.

With better information and a reflective mindset, you'll see your starting point, desired destination, and how to navigate obstacles effectively.

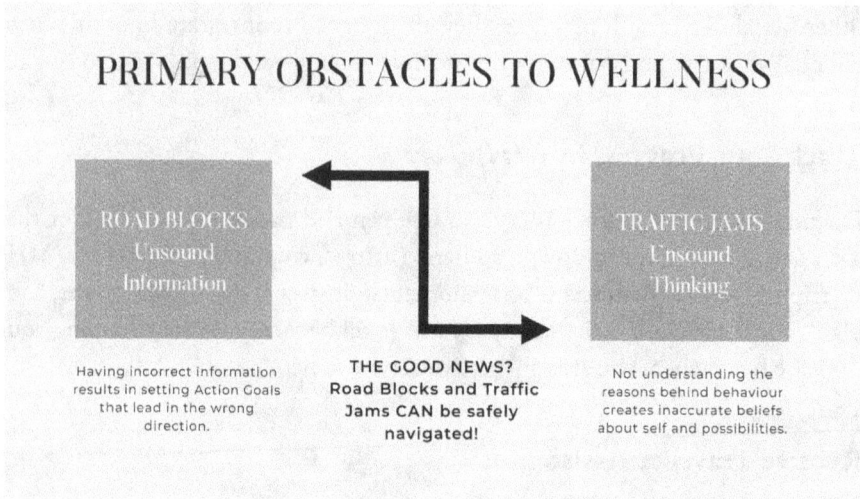

PRIMARY OBSTACLES TO WELLNESS

ROAD BLOCKS Unsound Information		TRAFFIC JAMS Unsound Thinking
Having incorrect information results in setting Action Goals that lead in the wrong direction.	**THE GOOD NEWS?** Road Blocks and Traffic Jams CAN be safely navigated!	Not understanding the reasons behind behaviour creates inaccurate beliefs about self and possibilities.

Primary Obstacles to Wellness

The Journey Ahead

This book equips you with essential strategies guided by decades of my experience in holistic nutrition, social work, and faith community leadership. However, I can't dictate your metabolic health journey—it's as individual as you, influenced by your background, body type, and personal experiences.

Gradually implement the steps and diligently follow through, and soon enough, your wellness destination will begin to appear on the horizon.

Let's Do This!

Prepare for simple, sensible, and science-supported steps to an epigenetical-ly-enhanced life. Expect strategies that promise significant results without over-whelming you, laying a foundation for lasting metabolic health.

TRIP ITINERARY

Information Centres

Clear, simple and relevant wellness material and practices, in bite-sized chunks (and with options, no less!).

Rest Stops

Questions to ask yourself and to journal answers. Then time to ponder what your body|mind|spirit thinks.

RoadWork

"Rubber meets the road" suggestions of how to put the *Leg's* information into action. Choose one!

Traveller Assistance

Here's where you'll find one suggested tool per *Leg* to make that section of the journey (and life!) go smoother.

Souvenirs

You'll want something to remember each *Leg* of the journey and to best prepare for what is around the corner.

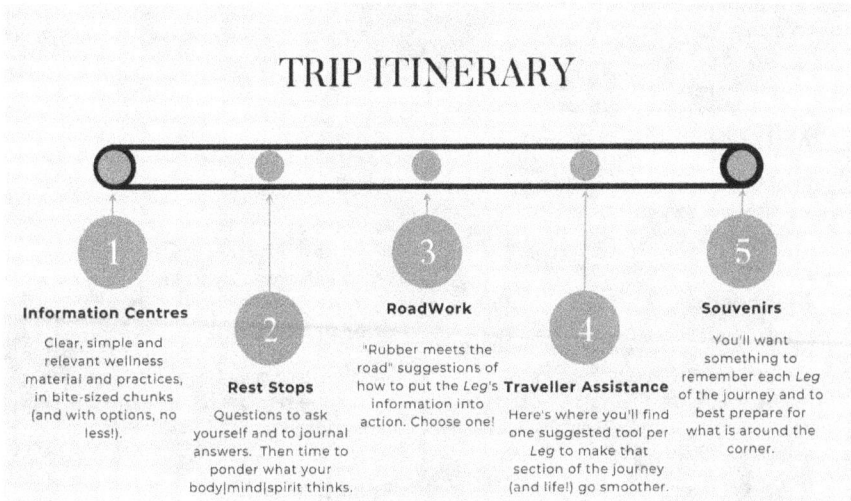

Metabolic Health Trip Itinerary

Ready to Start?

Take a peek at the glossary (of potentially unfamiliar terms or usage) that follows, and then get ready to embark on this "Metabolic Health Roadmap" journey to unlocking a healthier, more vibrant you. This isn't just about reading; it's about transforming—step by step, choice by choice.

Glossary

Action Goals (Clear Steps)

Specific, measurable steps that you alone can complete, they don't require the uncertain cooperation of someone else.

Diagnostics

Helpful assessment tools you'll find at the start of Legs 2-6, Diagnostics will help you assess your current levels of wellness and can be used, periodically in the future, to determine positive change.

Faith Goals (Dreams)

The vision or dreams as to where you are headed on the wellness journey. What you want to BE, DO, HAVE and GIVE.

BALANCE

An acronym for 7 essential components of wellness that are covered throughout the book. B-Balance, A-Attitude, L-Laughter and play, A-Activity, N-a good Night's sleep, C-Clean water and E-Eat for health.

Roadmap

A handy-dandy two page summary of the whole book, the Wellness Revolution Roadmap outlines key information from each Leg, helps you succinctly keep track of what's most important and asks pertinent questions that allow you to personalize your wellness plan for YOU.

Traffic Jams

Ways of thinking or believing that negatively impact your behaviour and ability to make healthful changes.

Energy Net Gains

Spending time and labour resources now and, later, getting a large wellness return on the investment!

Road Blocks

Wrong information (nutrition, fitness, sleep, stress management) that can lead to "stuckness" on the road to wellness.

Trip Log

This companion manual is recommended for use throughout your wellness journey.

Completion of the Trip Log will help you better learn, absorb more fully, and more consistently follow-through on information that you record and measure.

Set for Success Chart

The Set for Success Chart is your accountability-on-the-go tool. When you come to Leg 6, complete the chart for a baseline, and then regularly (I suggest once/month) for simple, accurate feedback.

Metabolic Health Roadmap Glossary

Chapter Two

LEG 1 - Five "W"s and a Love Letter

E arlier, I described metabolic health as including, among other things, adequate energy production and utilization.

When you strip wellness right back to its core, it is that energy—the ability of your cells to efficiently produce the power to drive your many bodily systems and functions—that largely determines your physical, mental, and emotional health.

A metabolically sound body breaks down food and utilizes nutrients to maximize energy flowing through a living system: YOU!

Therefore, in our discourse on metabolic health, we will primarily focus on improving eating, sleeping, moving, and calming methods to maximize energy production and free up vitality to keep you in a balanced state. We'll also focus on making those improvements in a personalized manner.

Once more, before we get started, if you haven't already, click here (https://www.inbalancelm.com/MHR_triplog) to download your copy of the *Trip Log*.

Leg 1 is pretty simple, with two main parts: the beginning of our road trip conversation (for which I wrote you a love letter) and 5 Wellness "W"s.

After you've read the letter and answered the Wellness "W" diagnostic questions, you can call it a wrap on your first leg of the journey. And on that note, let me welcome you to the Wellness Revolution. The Metabolic Wellness Revolution, that is. And in true road trip fashion, say:

Ladies and gentlemen, start your engines. Let the journey to eating, sleeping, moving, and calming for metabolic health begin!

Starting Our Road Trip Conversation

I LOVE what I do!

As a nutritionist and wellness coach, I am fortunate to work with people I like. People who are looking to grow physically healthier (have more energy and be fitter). Get sharper mentally (feel like they are bringing their "A" game to their work, studies, or relationships). Have balance in their emotions (experience deep joy, be present in deep grief, always with an underlying calm thread). Dig deeper into spiritual matters (become more generous and connected with themselves, others, and their sense of the sacred).

When I work 1-1 with clients, share in a small group setting, or teach hundreds on a Zoom call, some of that passion and enjoyment comes through. Clients and participants hear my excitement about bringing them the latest research, in the "nutshell" version most of them prefer.

They see my enthusiasm for supporting others in how I coach objectively and compassionately.

When we share a joke, or I pass along my latest favorite mindfulness reading, they glimpse my heart and my concern for their health and well-being.

How Can You Know That?

However, when I started writing this book, I was uneasy about conveying that passion and enthusiasm in the written word.

- How will you note how much I care about you if you don't hear the inflection of interest in my voice?

- How will you get how funny I am (or, according to my kids, *think* I am) if you can't see my exaggerated arm movements or catch the dramatic pause before a punch line?

- How will you know how much I've fervently researched the topics I'm about to share if you don't get to participate with me in a lively Q&A session?

"Write them a love letter!"

As I often do (and teach in this book), when uncertainty is swirling, I put out my questions—in this case, how to best communicate "me" to "you"—to the universe on a Rest Stop. (Feel free to use whatever term for "universe" works for you: the divine, God, common good, source, collective thought).

I "take a walk," but not just any old walk. A walk on the trails in my neighborhood, where I am surrounded by nature. Where I shut up and listen. No requests. No brainstorming. No to-do list creation. Just quietness.

Inevitably, I start hearing a few rumbles of answers. And on this day, as I was quietly present with how to best reach you, it came: "Write them a love letter."

Picture a raised eyebrow and a slightly quizzical shape to my mouth. A love letter, you say. To my readers? I couldn't, however, shake the idea. And the more I thought about it, the more sense it made. And so, your letter!

Dear Reader:

Thank you for being here. I appreciate you and everything it took for you to get here.

I see you. People buy this book for many reasons, but those reasons often include the fact that what they've been doing isn't working. I see that. I'm sorry. And I hope that that changes.

I care about you. I was once very sick. It's not a nice place to be. If you are not experiencing the physical, emotional, and mental health you long for, I can relate, and I wish more for you.

I have hope for you. Depending on how long you've wished for increased wellness and the number of diets, potions, exercise routines, supplements, mindfulness activities, and the latest/greatest "anything" you've tried, there is still an opportunity to learn, grow, and have things change.

Even if your hope quotient is low, know that after all the health ideas my clients and I have previously tried and where we're now wellness-wise, my hope levels hover high. I'm happy to loan you some of mine until yours can grow.

Finally, the word "love" itself. I don't use it lightly. I mostly reserve it for my immediate family members and close friends.

When I first thought of writing you a love letter, I immediately rejected it because of my value for the word and all that comes with it. But then I was reminded that there are many expressions of and meanings for the word "love."

Take the seven Greek meanings of love, for example (nope, I will not list them in the original language; I studied many things, but not Greek. I learned them by osmosis from my husband when he was getting his Master's in Theology!): empathy, friendship, romance, playfulness, self-love, commitment, and unconditional love.

Hear that this letter comes to you on the wings of the first love listed above—empathy. I like someone through the fondness of familiarity. I have a love for you forming because you are likely walking a journey with which I'm acquainted. I appreciate your courage. I value your willingness to change. My affection for you is already growing.

Love,

Brenda

The Five Wellness "W"s

As in all good detective work or creative writing, the classic five "W"s work excellently with metabolic health work, too!

Who?

Who are you? What's your current life situation? Everyone is in a different place on the journey. Reviewing these 5 "W"s and developing a doable plan that works for YOU is critical.

Now imagine discovering how to make that happen in less than three days (AKA doing two *Metabolic Health Roadmap* Legs a day over a long weekend) or on a 30+ day journey—your choice. Either works well!

What?

What does wellness look like to you? Can you draw a picture or create art to represent that wellness visually? Can you use words to describe the feelings you'll experience when optimal wellness is reached?

Have your downloaded *Trip Log* open and ready for sketching or taking notes.

When?

When are you going to schedule the time needed to become healthy? In the *Metabolic Health Roadmap*, I give you simple, sensible, sustainable tools to reach optimal wellness. Simple as they are, however, they will require at least a little time and energy expenditure on your part.

Look at your calendar and give yourself the gift of slotting in time for:

- Menu planning and meal and snack preparation.

- Choosing natural, fresh food.

- Discovering the fantastic uniqueness of your body type.

- Gentle (and some vigorous) movement in a manner that brings you joy.

- Rest, healing, and restoration.

- Stress management that suits your personality and life experiences.

You don't need many hours, but you do need a small amount of time. As one of my clients and now good friends, Angie, says, "Small choices made in the right direction will, over the years, change the trajectory of our lives in profound ways." Every decision you make, no matter how small, matters. Make room for that change.

Where?

Like in real estate, how well you succeed at your optimal wellness journey will require at least some attention to location, location, location.

In this case, it's not so much about the neighborhood where you'll purchase a house but, instead, where you want to go. Where do you see yourself in 3-5 years? Where will you be fitness-wise? Where will your mental health and clarity of mind be? Emotionally, where will you have landed? Where will you be spiritually in your relationship with the sacred or shared humanity?

Why?

At the top of the first page of your *Metabolic Health Roadmap Trip Log*, journal, or computer document, list at least one reason you are here.

There is a reason you bought this book, a reason you've set aside time to read it, a reason that has pushed you to improve your physical, emotional, and spiritual health.

What is it? You'll need it written down because you want to return to it at the beginning of each Leg. It will be your focus, underlying motivation, and why you will follow through with any relevant-to-you steps I suggest.

My *Why* for starting this journey was because, as you now know, I was a very sick and sad social worker. And I didn't want that to be the end of my story.

I loved my job, my marriage, and much of my life. Except for the fact that I had significant digestive issues, immune system challenges, thyroid problems, anxiety, insomnia, and, at the ripe old age of 25, I had developed an ulcer.

Where my *Why* took me was to become a healthy, energetic, and relatively sound-minded mom of five, grandmother of six (thus far), and partner of one pretty darn fantastic guy. Someone living a vibrant life of purpose that includes helping others live a vibrant life.

What's your *Why*, and where is it going to take you?

Wellness Revolution Roadmap

When you are doing the deep work of examining where you are headed, it can be nice to have that wellness journey roughed out for you. Thus, the Wellness Revolution Roadmap notes all six Legs along the way clearly and straightforwardly.

Everything is summed up in two graphics. Yup. Just two graphics! Take a look. It's all there! Skimmers can thank me later.

Wellness Roadmap - Part 1

Manage Stress for Energy

1) Notice what you are noticing
2) Evaluate what you need

☐ Bottom Up work to support the old/emotional brain (dance, massage, nature)
☐ Top Down work to support the newer/rational brain (yoga, meditation, mindfulness)

Don't forget to complete your Success Chart. It gives direction on where to start!

What are your primary stressors? Try to detect at least one in each body|mind|spirit category.

Move and Rest for Energy

Describe your new sleep hygiene routine. Include one each body | mind | spirit step.

Which of the 7 Primal Moves are you first going to incorporate?

Endless Energy for Life

What are the four Travel Destination Faith Goals? Things you would like to:

1 _____
2 _____
3 _____
4 _____

☐ In the travel-sized version of your Destination Plan you currently concentrate on BE and DO Faith Goals.

List five things you already do well and can use to Habit Hitch with new Action Goals. Pick one of each in the: eat, sleep, activity, attitude, and laughter & play categories.

1 _____
2 _____
3 _____
4 _____
5 _____

☐ I will ask questions of others (to gain knowledge/avoid Road Blocks), and of myself (to discover reasons for behaviours/dissolve Traffic Jams).

FINISH

Wellness Roadmap - Part 2

TRAVELLER ASSISTANCE

Wellness is a concept of the whole body, the whole mind, and the whole spirit. We're not a skin-enclosed container of isolated parts.

Improved metabolic health has the potential to enhance energy levels, reduce the risk of chronic disease, and facilitate reaching and maintaining a comfortable size.

There are significant links between metabolic health and improved cognitive function. A healthy metabolism provides a stable supply of nutrients and energy, which is vital for optimal brain functioning and can reduce the risk of neurode-generative diseases like dementia and Alzheimer's Disease.

Metabolic health also plays a role in our emotional and spiritual wellness. Well-regulated blood sugar levels (which a stable metabolism can help maintain) support mood stability and neurotransmitter regulation. Better energy management leads to better stress management.

Simply making environmental changes that improve metabolic health creates a positive feedback loop that ripples across physical, emotional, mental, and spiritual domains. While metabolic health is often first thought of as a collection of physiological processes in the body—which indeed it is—it can foster a holistic sense of wellbeing overall.

My "Famous" Broccoli Rubber Band Exercise

When I teach live, I often have participants bring a broccoli rubber band (those thick pink or blue elastic bands used in the produce department) to the workshop. I have them take their pen, and equal distance apart on the rubber band, write three words: BODY, MIND and SPIRIT.

I then have them envision a challenging event impacting one of those parts: a financial setback, losing a sibling far too early, or perhaps a period of disordered eating. I have them stretch the rubber band and visually note the ripple effect that moves through the other two of their parts.

Then, I have them envision an optimistic scenario. Maybe they are discovering a method of alleviating their headaches, experiencing deep emotional healing through trauma-informed counseling, or getting a better understanding of their optimal food plan.

Again, they stretch the rubber band. Again, they see a ripple effect. To achieve wellness (or at least discover the steps to begin moving in that direction), you have to look at and, hopefully, begin to nurture and integrate all your parts better.

That means body|mind|spirit work. There is no way around it. That means, throughout this book, I'll ask you to ponder and consider questions in all three areas.

SOUVENIR

I'm suggesting one last pause here before you get on the road. Get a "broccoli" rubber band (or substitute a blank note card); write the words "body," "mind," and "spirit" on it, and then take a deep breath.

Put the rubber band or note card somewhere you can easily see it throughout reading this book. You may have a lot on your plate in every part of your being. You don't have to tackle it all at once. We'll go slowly. Simply. And wherever you determine to start, whichever RoadWork most resonates with you, know that eventually, your efforts will produce positive benefits for ALL of you!

Chapter Three

LEG 2 – Eat for Metabolic Health

SUMMARY – Travel Size Version

Where in This Leg, You'll Discover Pretty Well Everything You Need to Know About Food and Drink!

L eg 2 is where you learn to eat for energy, health, and vitality. But first, we'll look at the keys to growth.

Essential Keys to Growth

1. Energy – What this book is about!

2. Clarity – Doing a complicated topic simply and clearly.

3. Structure – Where you are headed and the best way to get there.

4. Accountability – So you don't talk yourself out of what you say is important.

5. Feedback – Do the Leg Diagnostic tests and accept my free Wellness Roadmap Call offer!

Diagnostic #1 - BALANCE Wellness Wheel

You'll complete the BALANCE Wheel and see where you stand in seven critical wellness categories.

Three Food Foundations

When you can't remember anything else, come back to these three essentials:
- Eat real food.

- As close as possible to its original form.

- Don't fall prey to food fanaticism.

Five Food Keys

- Minimize refined foods (grains, sugars, highly processed seed oils).

- Eat enough protein (meat, poultry, fish, eggs, legumes, nuts and seeds).

- Get enough healthy fats (butter, olive and coconut oil, avocado, nuts and seeds).

- Watch the dairy (if dairy tolerant, eat cleanly sourced, modest amounts).

- Increase your vegetable intake (and, if tolerated, eat some fruit).

This Leg is where you look a little closer at what goes into your grocery cart (and, therefore, your mouth!) and grow in understanding of how essential nutrients and blood sugar regulation impact overall metabolic health.

Digging a Little Deeper

You'll also learn about Energy Net Gains (for example, expanding five minutes of smoothie-making into 15 freed-up mid-morning minutes of not being hungry), glean a ton of helpful information on cravings (and how to calm them!), discover my OCC (Objective, Curious, Compassionate) Action Plan for Self-Awareness, and get all your basic food information in a straightforward food pyramid.

Chapter Four

LEG 2 – Eat: Getting Started

"Opportunity without structure is chaos."

Keith J. Cunningham, The Road Less Stupid

During my decades of working with clients, workshop participants, parishioners (and myself!), I've learned a lot about how people grow. Gaining that insight has informed how I work and teach and is how I designed the *Metabolic Health Roadmap.*

Generally, in some form or other, I address and include five essential keys to growth and set those keys on a seven-component wellness framework of BALANCE.

The Five Essential Keys to Growth

Energy

More on this in a moment, as it's a biggie. In the meantime, if you don't have healthy cellular energy production (aka metabolic health), nothing much else—positive results-wise—in the book or your wellness journey will happen.

Clarity

"Wellness can be complicated. I make it simple. And doable. So you can be your best YOU!" A client came up with that. She looked at everything I've done with her and that I do in my practice and decided that should be my tagline (It was either that or Body Detective, and I was afraid if I chose that moniker, people might think I worked in police forensics and start calling me to help with cold cases!).

Structure

You need to know where you are headed and understand the framework that gets you there. Another word for structure is strategy. Strategy is the answer to overcoming the obstacles that keep you from reaching your wellness destination. However, it does need to be flexible and something you are excited about!

Accountability

Because, as one of my clients "infamously" said, "I can talk myself out of anything," how can we handle the accountability step, even from a distance?

It is more challenging to have accountability with readers than with clients I regularly meet in person, but here are some ways we can still achieve this.

- **Complete the Diagnostics found throughout the Legs.** At the end of the book, after you've finished all the exercises and come up with your Wellness Revolution Roadmap, you'll have an accurate picture of where you currently are, wellness-wise.

- **Be specific with the assessments.** Those metrics will help you measure how far and quickly you're moving toward your destination.

In addition:

1. **Journal:** Write down the action steps you completed that day.

2. **Prepare:** Know what you are doing tomorrow. Use your journal to write down several action steps for the days ahead. Take a lead from the information you'll learn below regarding Seed Habits.

3. **Measure:** What is measured is what gets done and what can be improved. Get insights from an upcoming Travellers Assistance on how to

Grow a Good Habit and Weed a Bad Habit.

4. **Share:** Let someone in on your game plan and set up a regular connection time. It will help you follow through on what you say is important to you.

Feedback

This essential change or growth component is the most complicated one to communicate between an author and a reader.

You can email me at info@inbalancelm.com to let me know how you are doing!

Even better is letting me know you'd like a free 20-minute <u>Wellness Roadmap Call,</u> during which we can examine where you've been, where you're headed, and what suggestions I'd make for increasing your health and wellness.

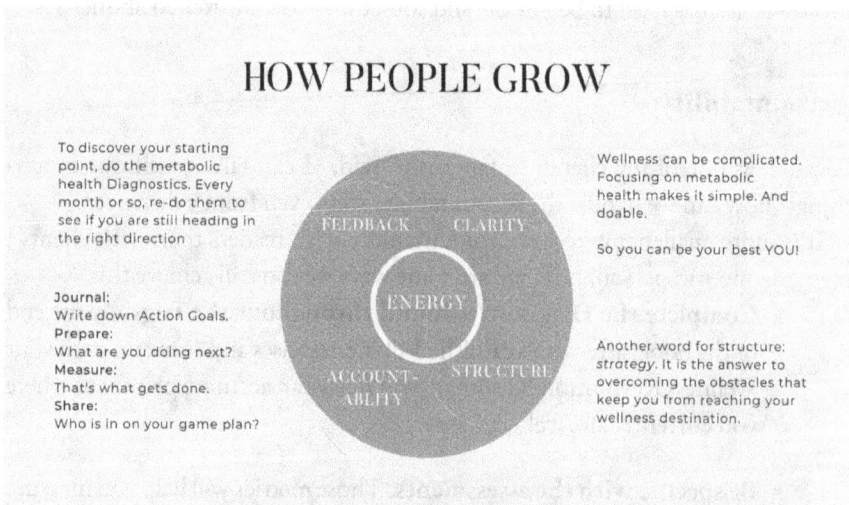

HOW PEOPLE GROW

To discover your starting point, do the metabolic health Diagnostics. Every month or so, re-do them to see if you are still heading in the right direction

Journal:
Write down Action Goals.
Prepare:
What are you doing next?
Measure:
That's what gets done.
Share:
Who is in on your game plan?

FEEDBACK   CLARITY

ENERGY

ACCOUNT-   STRUCTURE
ABLITY

Wellness can be complicated. Focusing on metabolic health makes it simple. And doable.

So you can be your best YOU!

Another word for structure: *strategy.* It is the answer to overcoming the obstacles that keep you from reaching your wellness destination.

How People Grow

In the meantime, understand that my first goal is to show you some destination options: more energy, a clearer mind, balanced moods, a greater sense of the "other," and a comfortable-for-you body size.

My next goal is to help you discover the Road Blocks (unsound information) and Traffic Jams (unsound thinking) on the road to that destination (get to the root of the problem). My final goal is to provide you with simple tools to move sensibly and sustainably from where you are to where you want to go.

You'll want to not only, as mentioned above, complete all the metabolic health Diagnostics (check-ups/tune-ups) but for additional feedback, you'll also want to periodically re-do some of the book's assessments (Wellness Wheel, BALANCE Success Chart) so that you can see if, down the road, you took a wrong turn.

Any positive shifts in your scores will show increased education, courage, and hope, which increases the likelihood of you following through on your wellness commitments. And that's great feedback to get at any time!

Diagnostic #1 - BALANCE Wellness Wheel

The seven components of wellness we'll examine throughout the book can be nicely summed up this way: B – Body type; A – Attitude; L – Laughter and play; A – Activity; N – a good Night's sleep; C – Clean water and Common good; and E – Eating for health.

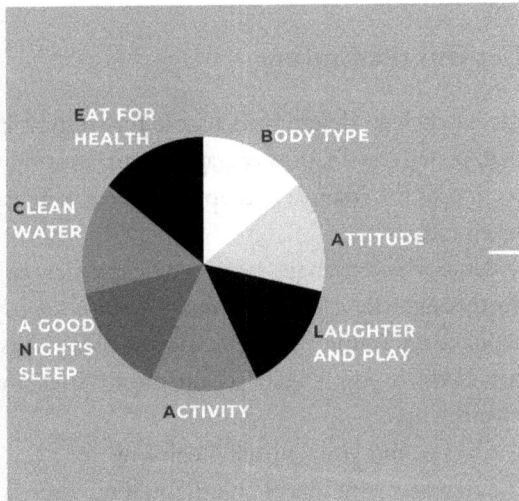

BALANCE WELLNESS WHEEL

On a scale of 1-10, rate yourself wellness-wise in each of the BALANCE categories (1 is low, 10 is optimal).

Once you've determined a score, using a felt pen or crayon, starting at the centre of the wheel, colour a section of the triangle that corresponds to your score in that category.

EAT FOR HEALTH • BODY TYPE • ATTITUDE • LAUGHTER AND PLAY • ACTIVITY • A GOOD NIGHT'S SLEEP • CLEAN WATER

BALANCE Wellness Wheel

Incorporate these seven components regularly into your lifestyle, and wellness will become reachable, easily attainable, and simple to restore when life throws you unexpected glitches.

Completing the BALANCE Wellness Wheel

On a scale of 0-10, 10 as the healthiest (and the outer edge of the circle), how well do you feel you are doing personally in each of the seven following areas:

- Body type

- Attitude

- Laughter and play

- Activity

- A good Night's sleep

- Clean water

- Eat for health

Take note, too, of your score in a less frequently considered "C" category, Common good (or, if you prefer, sense of Source or the Divine). While not officially noted on the Wheel, its threads are woven through the Attitude, Laughter and play, and a good Night's sleep Legs.

Get Out the Crayons

Once you have determined a score for yourself in each of the areas, using a felt pen, pencil crayon, or wax crayon, starting at the center of the wheel (0), color a section of the triangle that approximates your score in that area for each of the seven categories.

Note which triangles have significantly less color (and a lower score). As you go through the *Metabolic Health Roadmap,* pay the most attention to Road Blocks and Traffic Jams that address those areas. Working on those categories first is where you'll likely get the most "bang" for your labor, time, and money investment!

Oh yes, and give yourself "high fives" or a few minutes of "happy dance" for the triangles with lots of color! You'll use those areas for Habit Hitching (more on that later).

I'll Repeat It: Energy Trumps Everything

You'd think, as I'm an extremely analytical and linear thinker, we'd now begin with the first letter in the BALANCE acronym "B." But we are not because, remember, energy trumps everything.

For improved metabolic health and increased energy, you generally start by examining the type of fuel you're putting in your engine: Eating for health.

Chapter Five

LEG 2 - Three Food Foundations

"One of the very nicest things about life is the way we must regularly stop whatever it is we are doing and devote our attention to eating."
Luciano Pavarotti and William Wright, Pavarotti, My Own Story

INFORMATION CENTRE

I promised simple.

When standing in a grocery store aisle, perusing the menu at a restaurant, or scanning the plethora of options at your friend's overflowing New Year's Day buffet table, take a deep breath and remember these Three Food Foundations:

1. Eat real food.

2. As close as possible to its original form.

3. Don't fall prey to food fanaticism.

If you've ever heard me speak or have read any of my writing on nutrition, you may have previously heard me talk about the Three Food Foundations. You may be hoping that somewhere in my last batch of research, I've discovered new studies that have led me to change my nutritional cornerstones, preferably to something like 1) eat a lot of potato chips; 2) avoid anything that smacks of vegetable matter; and 3) be particularly zealous about upping your caffeine intake.

Sorry. That is not going to happen.

You'll hear the same Three Food Foundations over and over. That's because they're still science-supported. That science includes, very recently, a 2024 umbrella review of meta-analyses on ultra-processed food exposure and adverse health outcomes published in the British Medical Journal, showing that whole and minimally processed foods are the best way to support health.

That, in turn, means that following these three Food Foundations will help you reach your wellness destinations. They are still the best and simplest way I've found to live a healthy, balanced life (with, for many people, some room for chocolate!).

Food Foundation #1 – Eat Real Food

What I mean by "eat real food" is that if you genuinely want to be healthier, have more energy, be more clear-headed, have balanced moods, and reach and maintain a comfortable-for-you size, you need to eat things meant to be eaten. Preferably, they should be fresh and local (within a 10-100-mile radius).

Eating real food means minimizing "less than real" items: foodstuffs containing chemicals and additives like Splenda® and the dyes and preservatives found in items like colored or candy-coated breakfast cereals.

Avoid the excitotoxins (things that can potentially stimulate your brain's cells to death) such as MSG and Aspartame™. I don't know about you, but the more mature I get, the more protective I get of my brain cells. Not stimulating them to death resonates with me as a good action plan.

Eating real food means shopping on the outside edges of the grocery store (vegetables, fruits, meats, eggs, cheese) with only occasional forays into the middle aisles for things like olive oil, nuts, quinoa, or toilet paper.

That means the breakfasts you make, the lunches you pack, the snacks you grab, and the supper you cook in your home should primarily consist of foods available before World War II. Concentrate on meats, vegetables, fruit, and, for some people, safer starches like basmati or wild rice or millet instead of what has come to be known as "ultra-processed" foods: foods mainly composed of refined grains and sugars, with add-ons of edible oil by-products, dyes, and artificial flavoring.

Real Food, Real Simple

Eat the type of food your grandmother or great-grandmother would have consumed. Why real food? Because that is the fuel on which our bodies are best designed to function. You gain increased metabolic health on increased intake of real vs ultra-processed food. This point is critical when fueling for sports, work, or life stages like pregnancy, but it is vital at any time.

What You Eat Grows Your Body

In not-very-scientific terms, food gets chewed on, travels down the esophagus, is chemically attacked in the stomach, spewed into the small intestine, dragged through the intestinal lining, and then carried via the bloodstream to the liver, where it is recombined into the molecules needed to support healthy organs and systems. It bears repeating: What you eat grows your body!

Food Foundation #2 – Eat Food as Close as Possible to its Original Form

Food Foundation number two is also a fairly easily understood and applied principle. While I do not recommend eating raw, unwashed, freshly dug-up-from-your-garden potatoes, it is easy to see that a baked or roasted potato is closer to its "back to basics" beginnings, than its processed, poor-quality oil and chemical-added, preformed cousin, the Tater Tot!

Likewise, a slice of roast beef from a grass-fed, non-medicated, pastured, and ethically treated cow has a much better "back to basics" rating than a burger patty from an antibiotic-riddled, knee-deep in excrement housed, factory-farmed animal. (Sorry, that was a little graphic. If you've ever driven the I-5 down through California, however, and taken a big whiff—before coughing and gagging—of the air quality around the Fresno exit, you'll know what I'm talking about regarding the concern that factory farms might not be a good idea for cows, people or the pl anet.).

This foundation will be more or less challenging to fulfill depending on one's location, food budget, and the quality of food available. Simply be aware and do the best you can.

Concentrating on eating foods close to their original form leads us to the third Food Foundation.

Food Foundation #3 – Don't Fall Prey to Food Fanaticism

Due to today's refined food intake, our search for love and life in all the wrong places, and the psychological and physiological effects of some foods on our bodies, many North Americans have food or diet plan addictions. We don't eat to live, but rather, live to eat. And we often pendulum swing on what that living to eat looks like.

Full disclosure here. I mentioned I was a very sick social worker, with much of that being due to childhood illness. Probably an equally high factor, however, was my love of Peak Freen cookies and Nanaimo Bars (for those unfamiliar with the latter, Google it, and you'll understand!). Addiction would not be too strong a word to describe our relationship.

In the regional Family and Children's Services office where I worked, we had an "honor" box in the staff room. It was a cardboard box full of packaged baked goods (none of which would fall under the category of the first Food Foundation—real food). A little compartment in the corner of the box was where you'd insert your cash to purchase the sweet and sugary item calling your name.

When the vending company came to restock the snacks and collect the paid monies, saying I'd contributed much of my paycheck to the cause would not be an exaggeration. Food fanaticism at its finest.

Whether caffeine, sugar, the texture of crisp, fried foods, carbohydrates, chocolate, or _____ (you fill in the blank), hundreds of thousands of children and adults have lost the ability to make sound food choices and instead have let certain food items or food in general, become their fixation.

Let me say to you and my younger self: It's not your fault.

Food Foundation #3.5 – How You Eat is Not Entirely on You

Consider this a BONUS Food Foundation!

We're up against formidable Road Blocks (unsound info–spoiler alert: we'll be talking about Bliss Points in a future chapter), and most of us weren't raised with the tools to navigate the Traffic Jams (unsound thinking) safely.

As we better understand what we're up against food industry-wise and start looking to find our security and significance in worthier places, we can wean ourselves from the foods that have unhealthy holds on our minds and bodies.

The eventual outcome? Our ability to make good food choices returns, and with it, energy, clarity, balanced moods, comfortable-for-us body size, AND, for those of you with some form of staff room honor box in your life, the retention of more of your pay cheque!

On the other end of the food fanaticism spectrum are those for whom extremely healthy eating has become such a rigidly ingrained belief that they are unable to celebrate well on occasions where foodstuffs may contain a little sugar (provided they are not abstaining due to addictive responses) or where the offered food at a festive event does not meet their strict dietary guidelines.

That is also a position to avoid, or if you're already there, it is also likely not your fault. With the tools found in this book and, if needed, the work of an excellent trauma-informed therapist or a nutritionist who understands the concept I call "educated intuitive eating"—setting intuitive eating on a platform of whole food and sound thinking—gradually work your way back from the extreme to a more balanced place.

THREE FOOD FOUNDATIONS

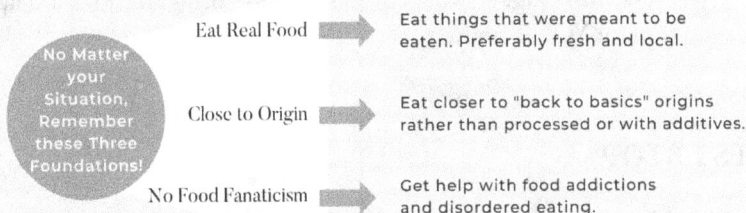

No Matter your Situation, Remember these Three Foundations!

Eat Real Food ➡ Eat things that were meant to be eaten. Preferably fresh and local.

Close to Origin ➡ Eat closer to "back to basics" origins rather than processed or with additives.

No Food Fanaticism ➡ Get help with food addictions and disordered eating.

Three Food Foundations

At either end of the food fanaticism spectrum, practice OCC: Objectivity (Hmmm, that's interesting!), Curiosity (I wonder what led me to believe that was a good idea?) and Compassion (Dang, girl, you were doing your best with the information you had; we can shift this!). I'll share more about my OCC–Action Plan for Self-Awareness in a future Traveller Assistance, but for the time being, this OCC, in brief, should help with Road Block or Traffic Jam exploration.

Once you are in a state of wellness where you feel good body, mind, and spirit and are comfortable in your skin and size, aim for an 80/20 position. That means about 80% of the time, you eat real food that suits your body type (more on that later, too) and makes you feel energetic, sleep soundly, and be calm and healthy, and about 20% of the time, you allow for "Sometimes" food and drink. These are foods or beverages that have no real physical benefit to health (and may, in fact, eaten in excess, contribute to illness) but that you choose, on occasion, to enjoy for celebratory or emotional reasons.

WHAT YOU'RE UP AGAINST:

- **Road Blocks:** advertising, Bliss Points, product placement in grocery stores, convenience.

- **Traffic Jams:** comfort foods, one-size-diet-fits-all beliefs, equating foods with reward.

TOOLS AT YOUR DISPOSAL:

- **New behaviors:** better-for-YOU shopping and cooking skills, ingredient awareness.

- **New thinking:** a "what else besides food brings me joy" list, appreciation for YOUR body.

REST STOP

Time to take a break and digest information! Per the diagram that follows, take 10 minutes of calm to Rest with the following questions:

1. Where am I on a healthy eating scale of 1-10 (With one being I wouldn't know a vegetable if it hit me in the head, and I think Combo #6 at my favorite fast-food joint is one of the four food groups, and ten being my backyard is a full-scale mini-farm, I make my cheese, and the herbal tea I'm drinking was personally dried in my kitchen!)?

2. Where do I already walk out the three Food Foundations well?

3. Where could I do a better job of following the Food Foundations? (In your *Trip Log*, draw a line down the center of a page. On the left side, list what you are doing well: eating real food as close as possible to its original form and not falling prey to food fanaticism. On the right side, make note of things you could improve.)

Next, Stop for 10 minutes of quiet (sitting or slowly walking). Keep your mind as clear and open as possible, and just listen. Jot down any responses that may arise. Because you've taken time to ponder calmly and quietly, these responses will most likely be less off-the-cuff and from a deeper level. They can give you clues as to the reasons behind your answers! Those clues, in turn, will reveal some of the Traffic Jam thinking and can provide great direction on moving forward!

REST STOP

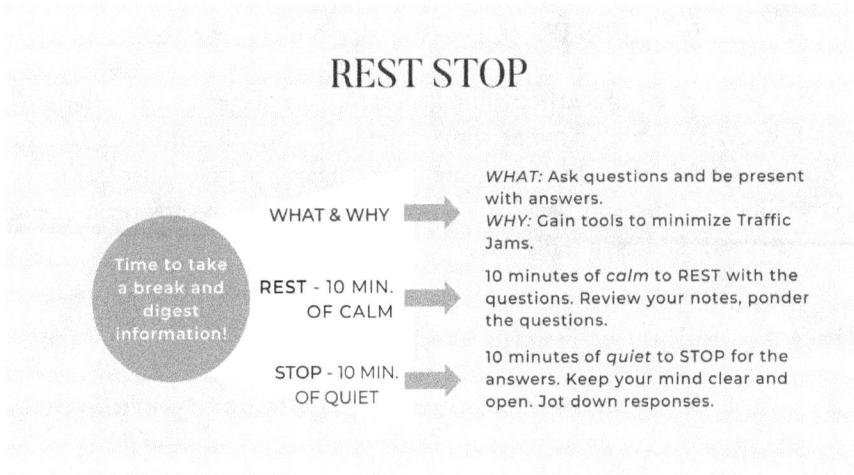

Time to take a break and digest information!	WHAT & WHY	*WHAT:* Ask questions and be present with answers. *WHY:* Gain tools to minimize Traffic Jams.
	REST - 10 MIN. OF CALM	10 minutes of *calm* to REST with the questions. Review your notes, ponder the questions.
	STOP - 10 MIN. OF QUIET	10 minutes of *quiet* to STOP for the answers. Keep your mind clear and open. Jot down responses.

Rest Stop

ROADWORK

This section is not just theoretical but is designed to guide you in choosing the most relevant option for your wellness journey. Choose the option that most resonates with you. Note the option and your response in your *Trip Log*.

Option 1 – Guesstimate how many items in your usual grocery store shopping cart are "real food" and how many are not. Write down the approximate percentages of each. Set an action step to gradually increase—by about 10% a trip—the percentage of real food each time you shop.

Realize that this will entail putting some packaged food back on the shelf—about 10% each week—and spending more time in the produce department and other sections on the perimeter of most grocery stores.

Option 2 – Begin to evaluate the resources needed for your wellness journey. Reflect on the time required for grocery shopping, chopping, and cooking. Acknowledge the effort that will be exerted as you take different action steps. And be sure to read the Traveller Assistance for this section of Leg 1. That's where you'll learn about Energy Net Gains to better understand the real value and eventual return of those expenditures.

Trouble getting started? Here's a question to prime the brainstorming pump: What do you need to spend less on to free up cash flow to buy higher-quality food? Remember to factor in the gains made dollarwise as you minimize or eliminate ultra-processed food purchases.

TRAVELLER ASSISTANCE – Energy Net Gains

Though we are all integrated body|mind|spirit parts, we'll spend most of the book on the body. The reason why? Starting with physical health generally offers the greatest potential to create the most significant increase in physical energy (back to metabolic health again!), which, in turn, will allow you to subsequently and more efficiently address mind|spirit concerns.

Once Again: Energy Trumps Everything!

When we calculate what it costs us to gain energy (E), we often get the equation wrong. That means we are reluctant to spend our finite resources of time (T), labor (L), and money (M) for what we might see as a poor return on the investment.

We ask ourselves if $1T + 1L + 1M$ will get us $3E$. Will I get 15 minutes of increased energy if I spend five minutes making breakfast with ingredients that cost me $5.00 and take medium-level physical exertion and brain power?

What if we're asking the wrong question, however? What if time, labor, and money weren't directly translatable into energy, at least not initially? What if it did take a little more out of you the first couple of times you tried a post-dinner walk or a noon time 10 minutes of mindfulness?

But then, what if, in a spin on the classic Jim Croce song, you actually could save energy in a bottle? And what if some of your activities that took time, labor, and money began returning double or triple the investment?

Saving Energy in a Bottle

- Five minutes to make a smoothie. Fifteen minutes net gain, not needing to go through a drive-through for coffee and a muffin when your energy tanks mid-morning. (Bonus? You saved on another resource: money!)

- Ten minutes on lunchtime mindfulness solitude. Thirty minutes net gain as you, then, quickly and with concise clarity, write up a kick-butt quarterly report.

- Thirty minutes on a post-dinner neighborhood walk. Two hours net gain in calm conversations with your teen pushing for a later curfew and your mom, who has finally decided she is ready to tour a couple of extended care homes.

As you read this book, you can pick up a few innovative health tools and spend some time learning how to minimize wellness Road Blocks and Traffic Jams. Like any new skill set, walking out those discoveries will take extra time and labor initially (along with the bucks it costs to buy this book!).

But, let me add, by getting that practice down pat, the potential to have more than enough energy to walk out every Leg of your wellness journey—to say nothing of efficiently accomplishing everything that awaits at your destination—will go through the roof.

Call it new math :). Know it will be easier than helping your 10-year-old with theirs!

Chapter Six

LEG 2 – Five Food Keys

"You eat peas and apples. And you make other people eat them, too!"
A kindergarten student, when I posed the following question
to her class: "Do you know what a nutritionist does?"

N ote: Her answer was so great I considered making it my business tagline!

INFORMATION CENTRE

Once you have the Three Food Foundations in place, add the Five Food Keys, and you will be well on your way with Nutrition 101 strategies. Putting them in place can create significant wellness in many areas. But the most pertinent thing at this point is that you'll better balance blood sugar levels, experience greater metabolic health overall, and feel a gradual increase in energy.

Once that happens, you'll not only have the stamina to climb over Road Blocks but should also begin to see an increase in the mental sharpness needed to examine the thinking leading to some of your Traffic Jams.

Food Key #1 – Minimize Refined Foods (Notably Ultra-Processed Sugar and Grain)

As a writer, I find it intriguing that a word like "refined" comes across as such an elegant word. One that could be descriptive of foods that I, as a nutritionist, would be encouraging you to include in a healthy diet. Nothing could be further from the truth! In reality, in food industry terms, the refining process is a series of steps that strip nutrients from natural foods and leave them as foodstuffs deficient in naturally occurring vitamins, minerals, and fiber. You're left with foodstuffs where their intake can play significant roles in declining metabolic health.

Depending upon your genetic responses to carbohydrates (we are all a little different in that regard), your intake of grains and sugar, in general, and particularly of ultra-processed grains and sugars, can impact your blood sugar levels, your insulin sensitivity, and even your risk for conditions such as metabolic syndrome and type 2 diabetes.

According to information from organizations such as the American Heart Association, Harvard School of Public Health and the World Health Organization, processed grain and sugar intake can contribute to:

Increased risk of insulin resistance and type 2 diabetes: When our intake of ultra-processed foods is too high for our tolerance levels, we can experience elevated blood glucose and insulin levels. Over time, this pattern can overtax the pancreas, potentially contributing to insulin resistance and, again, potentially being a factor in developing type 2 diabetes.

Overweight and obesity: Not in everyone, but for some, because refined sugars are highly caloric and are often included in the foods that have a high bliss point—more on that to follow—they have the potential to lead to excess weight gain and obesity.

Negative impact on lipid profile: For some, a high refined sugar intake can increase triglyceride levels and decrease high-density lipoprotein (HDL) cholesterol, potentially contributing to cardiovascular disease.

As we'll discuss shortly, it is not solely the higher carbohydrate intake typically found in ultra-processed foods that is of concern; some folks, after all, do pretty well on a higher carbohydrate intake. Along with worries over higher refined sugar and grain content, though, is concern about the unhealthy fat ingredients (refined polyunsaturated and trans fats), low fiber content, and poor nutrient quality of these foods.

Wherever you look—the British Medical Journal, Public Health Nutrition, or the Journal of the American College of Cardiology—it seems clear that reducing ultra-processed food consumption can substantially improve overall metabolic wellness.

Where We've Come From

Several generations ago, a family's dietary intake was grown or hunted locally and eaten in a whole food (unprocessed, non-medicated) form. Even the term processed was primarily reserved for methods like fermentation, sprouting, drying, or preserving. With advances in knowledge and expertise, the ability to separate and remove components of grain, fruit, or vegetables meant longer-term food storage became a reality.

Sugar cane and beets could undergo a 10+ step process, be stripped of everything but a few chemical molecules, and end up as virtually "last forever" bleached white sucrose crystals.

New equipment in flour mills allowed millers to remove the germ and bran—the outer, more easily spoiled grain components. The flour now had a longer shelf life and could be stored, transported, and sold to a broader market.

Even for those who digest grains well, this new product was less nutritious, though white flour had several vital factors going for it. Because it was new and less common, it was seen as somewhat of a status symbol (Witness the joy of us kids growing up in my family of origin when my parents were able to afford store-bought white bread and my mom no longer had to bake the heartier loaves none of us realized was more nutrient-dense!). Because of its longer shelf life, increased technology, and factory-produced foods, refined flour became the industry standard for processed items.

Convenience Comes at a Cost

The past 70+ years' worth of increased consumption of refined grains and sugars have contributed to a loss of essential nutrients, which in turn led to ailments including obesity and digestive disorders.

Excessive refined sugar and grain intake can cause fatigue, weight gain, arthritis, and depression in the short term. In the long term, potential ailments include dental cavities, heart disease, yeast overgrowth, hypertension, and hypoglycemia. Moving these foods to a rare Sometimes Food appearance (more on that to come) can improve metabolic health, reduce risk factors for many chronic illnesses, and foster an overall healthier life.

Food Key #2 – Eat Enough Protein-Rich Food

In the next section of this Leg of your wellness journey, we'll unpack the macronutrients—protein, carbohydrates, and fats—more thoroughly, but for starters, know that in my experience, upon completion of an initial tracking log, most of my clients discover they eat too many carbohydrate-rich foods (grains, cereals, bread, pasta, crackers, sugars, potatoes, rice and, perhaps, fruit) in proportion to protein-rich foods (red meat, chicken, lamb, turkey, fish, legumes, nuts, seeds, eggs, cheese). Even most food charts emphasize eating large amounts of grain-based foodstuffs at the expense of sufficient recommendations for protein foodstuffs, particularly for those with a Protein Body Type (another topic for a future Leg).

Start with Snack Time, Then Tackle Breakfast

Often, a simple way to help transition from too many grains is by addressing snack-time food options. Rather than having corn chips and salsa or crackers for a mid-afternoon snack, grab a healthy trail mix (real food, no candy bits, not too much dried fruit) and baby carrots or hummus and red pepper strips.

Next, start your morning with a natural, no-added-sugar yogurt, protein powder-based smoothie, or a couple of eggs. Or, if you tolerate grains well, enjoy nut butter on sourdough or sprouted whole-grain toast.

Even if you are physically active, perhaps training for a ½ marathon or going into a weekend pickleball tournament, fueling up on carbohydrates or "carb loading" is not generally recommended. A modest amount of carbohydrate-rich food (fruit, starchy vegetables, a few gluten-free nut and seed crackers) can be helpful, especially for body types that do better on higher amounts of carbohydrate-rich foods. Still, that must be coupled with small but regular amounts of protein-rich and fat-rich foods.

Food Key #3 – Get Enough Healthy Fat

"Hold it," you might say, "I thought a holistic approach to metabolic health would have me cutting fat from my diet." And in some ways, you are right. The unnatural, altered, chemically processed fats like the trans fats found in many French fries, chips, donuts, snack foods, salad dressings, margarine, and crackers should be minimized or eliminated. They are not in the proper form to be helpful to the body, and, much like putting a square peg in a round hole, they create havoc as the body tries to make do with them for the many essential roles that fats play i n wellness.

Trans fats are a type of unsaturated fat (usually liquid at room temperature) that has been chemically altered (the addition of hydrogen molecules to the carbon chain of unsaturated fats) to remain solid at room temperature. Think of a salad dressing that maintains emulsion without shaking and peanut butter, where you don't have to stir in the top layer of oil before making that tasty sandwich.

The hydrogenation process increases shelf life and product stability but also negatively impacts how fats are metabolized in the body, leading to increased insulin resistance, inflammation, and heart disease risks.

However, specific fats and fat-rich foods with a long history of traditional use play an essential role in metabolic health. They are necessary and of great benefit and should be eaten daily. This means regularly including foods like butter, olive oil, coconut oil, avocados, and, perhaps, fish oils, as well as nuts and seeds, in your diet.

Minimize or avoid heavily processed oils (soybean, canola, corn, sunflower, margarine).

Food Key #4 – Watch the Dairy Intake

And by that, I don't mean get your 6-8 servings of dairy/day. I'm not a huge fan of most dairy products (If they were still running the milk mustache ads, you wouldn't see my smiling face featured!). How dairy is produced today and—depending on where the milk is obtained, the potential of antibiotics or growth hormone residue—can contribute to challenges for kids, teens, and adults, including issues like allergies, asthma, eczema, acne, and ear infections.

Provided you are dairy-tolerant (no bloating, skin issues, or lactose or casein intolerance), my suggested nutritional approach allows for modest amounts of cleanly sourced dairy products as part of your daily protein-rich food intake. Cheese and yogurt are excellent protein sources for many people and can play a part in a health-supportive diet.

Dairy Intolerances

Just under 70% of the world's population cannot easily digest cow's milk. If you are in the minority and can eat dairy products, look for clean sources and, when available, choose organic options. If you have allergies or intolerances to dairy products, keep them out of your diet and instead, if desired, substitute other types of milk, yogurt, and cheese (almond or coconut).

Note that soy wasn't a recommended dairy substitute. While some people can benefit from soy's protein and other plant compounds (minerals and isoflavones, for example), soy is not necessarily helpful for everyone. Soy is one of the most commonly genetically modified crops and can also be difficult for people to digest. If you are soy-tolerant, eat soy in moderation and choose organic, fermented, and minimally processed forms.

Food Key #5 – Eat a Lot of Vegetables and a Bit of Fruit

Fresh vegetables and fruits are valuable sources of various vitamins, minerals, and enzymes and contain a variety of phytochemicals (plant chemicals) that play an essential role in disease prevention and eradication.

In their antioxidant role, vegetables and fruits help the body neutralize the damage caused by free radicals—enemies of good health produced by stress, toxins, and natural body processes.

Research also indicates that specific plant food properties help regulate the body's blood vessel growth correctly, ensuring that fat cells do not become too well-fed and thus grow more rapidly than they should.

Fresh produce also contains high water content, valuable fibers, and enzymes—catalysts for many of the body's metabolic processes. For those who are vegetable-tolerant, who don't, for example, need to avoid oxalates and the many vegetables that contain them, a wide variety of vegetables should be consumed in relatively high amounts daily, both raw and cooked (5-7 servings/day or even more if you enjoy them).

Commonly eaten varieties like carrots, cucumbers, and peas are a great start, but for maximum energy and wellness, include lots of dark leafy greens and cruciferous vegetables like cauliflower, kale, and broccoli. The latter can be eaten cooked by pretty well everyone, and depending upon detoxification genes, consumed raw for those who need to speed up their Phase 1 detoxification. Not sure of your detoxification genes? Stick mostly to cooked cruciferous vegetables and avoid greens products that contain raw cruciferous vegetables in the ingredients (i.e. broccoli sprouts). Consider occasionally substituting root vegetables such as sweet potatoes, parsnips, or yams for the potato, which is often overrepresented on the dinner table.

Where does fruit intake factor into a suggested wellness plan? Depending upon body type and dietary phase (and by that, I mean, are you trying to reduce candida levels? Are you on more of a Ketogenic plan?), 1-3 servings of fruit can also be eaten daily.

As much as possible, eat fruit that grows locally (for me, that is berries over mango) and choose whole fruit more often than fruit juice. The additional fiber in whole fruits contributes to good health, including slowing the metabolism of the fructose (fruit sugar) naturally contained in fruit.

FIVE FOOD KEYS

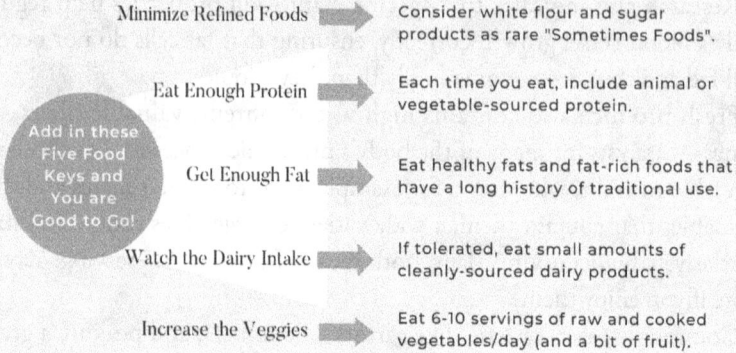

Minimize Refined Foods →	Consider white flour and sugar products as rare "Sometimes Foods".
Eat Enough Protein →	Each time you eat, include animal or vegetable-sourced protein.
Get Enough Fat →	Eat healthy fats and fat-rich foods that have a long history of traditional use.
Watch the Dairy Intake →	If tolerated, eat small amounts of cleanly-sourced dairy products.
Increase the Veggies →	Eat 6-10 servings of raw and cooked vegetables/day (and a bit of fruit).

Add in these Five Food Keys and You are Good to Go!

Five Food Keys

REST STOP

Time to take a break and digest information!

Take 10 minutes of calm to Rest and journal with the following questions:

1. What shopping and food prep skills do I need to develop to better eat for health?

2. Which foods do I want to minimize, and which do I want to increase?

Next, Stop for 10 minutes of quiet (sitting or slowly walking). Keep your mind as clear and open as possible, and just listen. Jot down any responses that may arise.

ROADWORK

Choose the option that most resonates with you. Note the option and your response in your *Trip Log*.

Option 1 – Head to your kitchen (or, if you're not near your kitchen, think about what is in your kitchen) and list the different types of vegetables and fruit in your fridge or freezer, on the counter, or in the pantry. Note both the name of the vegetable or fruit and the color. If tomorrow is shopping day, and the cupboards look bare, you get some grace. Make a list of what would generally be and will be there again once you return from the grocery store.

List made? How is it looking for variety? Lots of different types of vegetables and fruit? Are a wide range of colors represented? If so, keep it up. If not, you know an area for improvement on your next shopping trip.

Option 2 – Think about your food cravings and where they most likely originate. Jot down your responses. Then head to the next section, Traveller Assistance on Calming Cravings-ACDC Style, and read through the four main factors that can give rise to cravings.

Then, re-consider the original question. Knowing what you now know, from where do you think your cravings primarily originate? List one Action Goal you can put in place to avoid craving Road Blocks more easily.

TRAVELLER ASSISTANCE – Calming Cravings-ACDC Style

[This is a long Traveller Assistance. It's in response to how many of my clients—and how long I—dealt with cravings. Feel free to skip over this section if you don't have food or beverage cravings!]

No, I'm not much of an ACDC fan (their song lyrics don't generally align with my philosophies on life and relationships, although I do have a "fun fact" connection to the band in that our family is friends with close relatives of one of the band's drummers!), but the letters in their name make a great acronym for better understanding and dealing with food cravings.

Addiction. Culture. Deficiency. Chatter.

ADDICTION – When food and drink call your name, a lot!

When you are looking at cravings stemming from food intolerances or allergies, there are two primary ways that addiction can factor into those cravings. First, an example of how a substance to which one has an intolerance or allergy can become an addiction.

Opiate responses – Dairy products are one of the top ten foods to which people have allergies or intolerances. That allergy or intolerance can appear in many ways, including acne, eczema, and behavioral challenges. Even without apparent negative responses to dairy, it can be challenging for someone to break what is often a solid "love affair" with it. Here's one potential reason why.

Dairy protein—casein—has naturally occurring opiate molecules, some of which appear as casein fragments called casomorphins, a casein-derived morphine-like compound. When eaten, these fragments can attach to the same brain receptors to which heroin and other narcotics attach. Why that response? Maybe to ensure the survival of the species? For sure, the cow species, but as breast milk contains casein similar in structure to that in cow's milk, perhaps it's to ensure human babies enjoy and continue to nurse and foster the survival of our species as well. For those who love dairy products in cheese form, be aware this potentially addictive compound is concentrated about seven-fold in cheese. Even for individuals who would gladly be featured in a cheese mustache ad and have—like many people, no apparent negative reaction to casomorphins—note that the fat and salt content can still produce a plethora of "eat more of me" responses (more on this under Bliss Points in the Culture section coming up n ext).

Next, an explanation of how dopamine responses happen so you better understand why certain foods—chocolate or potato chips, for example—can become an integral part of that response.

Dopamine responses – Dopamine is a type of neurotransmitter. Your body makes it, and your nervous system uses it to send communication between nerve cells. That's why it's sometimes called a chemical messenger. Among other tasks, dopamine plays a role in our pleasure, motivation, and focus responses, and in the animal kingdom, it is a large part of our uniqueness as humans in thinking and planning.

What responses? Dopamine is released when your brain is expecting a reward. When you associate a particular activity with pleasure, mere anticipation may be enough to raise dopamine levels. What types of activities? Well, realistically, anything you might enjoy (shopping, sex, dancing), but pertinent here, eating a particular food. If a food has become "hardwired" into a dopamine response (pleasant memories, blood sugar rise with resulting energy and mood lift), untangling that connection by taking action such as choosing another activity from your "What Brings Me Joy?" list, having a power nap, doing a minute of jumping jacks, taking a supplement containing L-tyrosine (a building block for creating dopamine) or meditation or counseling, may be necessary to weaken the craving l ink.

Be aware, too, that dopamine responses happen with all kinds of foods (primarily ultra-processed ones), whether or not there are allergies or intolerances to that food.

CULTURE - What are we seeing, hearing, and being led to do?

I'll keep this short, as whole books could be and have been written on the impact of culture on our choices. So we'll stick with the biggies: advertising, food subsidies, and bliss points.

Advertising – Think online and print magazines; audio, TV, and streaming commercials; and where food is placed in grocery stores. Everything is designed to attract you (biggest promotion) to what manufacturers will profit from most (biggest markup).

Food Subsidies – Data compiled by 24/7 Wall St. (who, in turn, looked at data compiled by the Environmental Working Group, National Grower's Assoc., U.S. Census Bureau, the U.S. Department of Agriculture, and other organizations to determine changes in consumption over the past fifteen years) showed that producers of these products can be appropriately called the firms that benefit the most from U.S. farm subsidies (government financial aid supplied to farmers and industry).

In "Top 9," order from least to most subsidy (least is relative!): 9. sunflower oil; 8. peanuts; 7. ground beef; 6. milk; 5. sorghum/barley (animal feed, beer production); 4. rice; 3. soybean oil; 2. bread; 1. corn (some for corn-based ethanol, an alternative gas source; corn is also, however, one of the most consumed grains).

• Think about why free-range eggs, raspberries, and broccoli didn't make the list.

Bliss Points – Bliss point is a term coined by US market researcher and psychoanalyst Howard Moskowitz. The processed food industry uses it in engineering the formulations of three critical ingredients—salt (found in relatively high amounts in milk), sugar (found in corn syrup, grain, bread, and milk), and fat (found in sunflower oil, peanuts, soybean oil, and milk)—to deliver just the right amount of palatability to achieve the hedonistic pursuit of food, independent of hunger levels.

- Salt, sugar, and fat: Take note of the foods in the top subsidized products list that make the bliss points list. Are you starting to understand why I said some of your food choices and fatigued, brain-fogged, or moody gridlock in Traffic Jams are not your fault?

- Hedonistic pursuit of food: We've evolved to preferentially prefer just the Goldilocks-style "right amount" of these three salty, sweet, and rich flavors, and we pursue these pleasures because we love the endorphin hit we get when we eat them.

- Independent of hunger levels: Well-calculated bliss points overrule our "I think I'm full" messages and foster mindless eating! And you thought "Betcha can't eat just one!" was simply a catchy slogan.

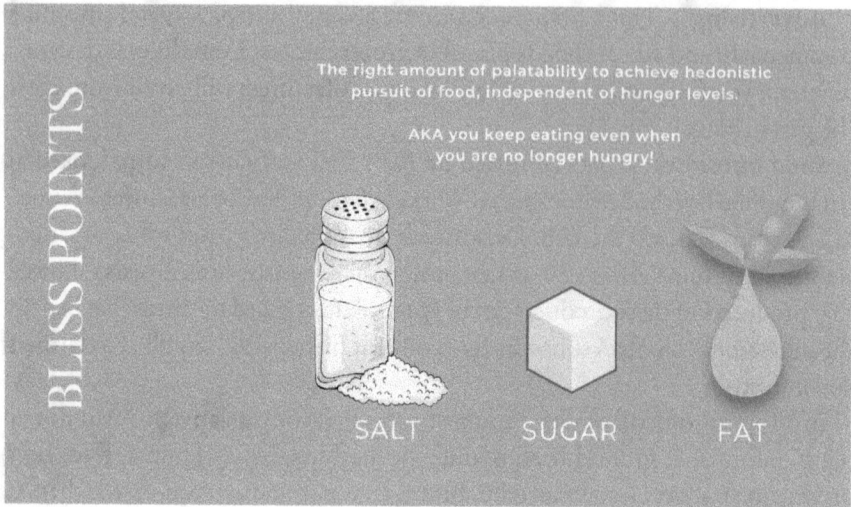

The right amount of palatability to achieve hedonistic pursuit of food, independent of hunger levels.

AKA you keep eating even when you are no longer hungry!

BLISS POINTS

SALT   SUGAR   FAT

Bliss Points

DEFICIENCIES – Primary Deficiencies Related to Cravings

There are many nutritional deficiencies that can contribute to cravings. Here are some of the primary possibilities.

Blood sugar fluctuations – While not a true deficiency, poor blood sugar regulation—often a result of poor diet and insufficient movement—can lead to more extreme blood sugar fluctuations throughout the day that, in turn, can produce intense carbohydrate cravings. Eating sugar or refined grains is the fastest way to bring them up again when blood sugar levels drop. To combat extreme fluctuations, eat whole foods for your body type (next Leg of the journey) and get regular, enjoyable exercise (also in a future Leg).

Specific nutritional deficiencies – For specific cravings, see if the following suggestions help. In all cases, note that a variety of real food options, including a wide range of different-colored vegetables, is a great place to start.

- Craving **sweets**? Get more magnesium, chromium, and tryptophan in your diet. These nutrients are found in whole foods, such as broccoli, dried beans, liver, eggs, poultry, legumes, and grains, or you can get them via supplementation.

- Craving **bread** may indicate a nitrogen deficiency; eat more fish, meat, and beans.

- Craving **fatty foods** may indicate you are not getting enough calcium. This mineral is found in seafood, dairy products, and leafy greens.

- Craving **chewing ice** may indicate a lack of iron in your diet. Eat leafy greens, fish, chicken, and black cherries to combat this craving.

- Craving **red meat** may indicate an iron deficiency. Check with your healthcare professional (as with all suspected deficiencies) to determine if this is true and, if so, follow their counsel along with eating leafy greens, fish, chicken, and black cherries.

CHATTER – "Body, Brain and Heart" Noise

For many of my clients, chatter is the most insidious and deeply entrenched factor contributing to food cravings.

Physically – as mentioned in the other three letters of the ACDC acronym, cravings, and their chatter can be a physical response to refined foods, nutritional deficiencies, and neurotransmitters or neurotransmitter-like compounds. Body cravings are great at calling our name loudly and at length!

Mentally – Brain Chatter often piles right on top of Body Chatter.

- **Monkey Brain:** When we experience an inability for our brain to easily quiet and rest, food can sometimes be used to reduce that anxiety.

- **Disordered Eating:** This can originate as trauma from our family of origin or outside-of-home adverse events. As Dr. Gabor Maté, a renowned addiction expert with a particular interest in childhood development and trauma, wisely stated, "Trauma is not what happens to you, it's what happens inside you as a result of what happened to you." Disordered eating can be a result; trauma-informed therapy with a skilled practitioner can help.

Emotionally – If food were only meant to keep us alive and came with no heartstrings attached, cravings would be a minor bump in the road to wellness. There are many links, however, between food and emotion or Heart Chatter. Some examples:

- **Parental challenge #1:** Though this historical concept is changing, fathers are typically seen as the protector or provider in a family. If either parent did not cover that role as you were growing up, then intake of particular foods or food, in general, can become seen as a shield of protection.

- **Parental challenge #2:** In many cultures, nurture, and comfort have often come in the arms of one's mother. If neither parent could offer consistent or sufficient nurture, certain baked goods, beverages, or favorite family dishes can genuinely become "comfort" foods.

- **Siblings/Friends challenges:** If you lacked the companionship of siblings or peers or experienced bullying or ostracization while growing up, food can play a friendship role.

Spiritually – I promised that throughout this book, I'd weave in threads of "common good," the divine, or what is beyond simply our physical and mental state. Note, therefore, that Body, Brain, and Heart Chatter can ripple spiritually as well. Negative self-talk or behaviour can impact our self-worth and sense of purpose.

That, in turn, can distort our relationships with others (our belief in their value or innate goodness) and with what links us as humans (the divine, source, common humanity). Cravings can be a symptom of deeper issues of one's significance and security.

While there can be much to attend to, cravings-wise, taking it step-by-step and layer-by-layer usually produces good results. If this ACDC Traveller Assistance resonates significantly with you, note that in Leg 6, I'll share a few more suggestions to help you deal with cravings. However, if the topic feels somewhat overwhelming, it is often best sorted out in a group, one-on-one consultation, or counseling. Please be open to following up on that if needed.

BONUS TRAVELLER ASSISTANCE – In BALANCE Food Pyramid

When a Food Photo is Worth 1000 Food Words!

Let's sum things up from the first two Legs with a graphic! This is where you'll see the food and wellness guidelines I created to reflect better how my family, my clients, and I get and stay healthy, a BALANCEd food pyramid designed to better support all of us in optimizing metabolic health!

All in one place. Easy, peasy.

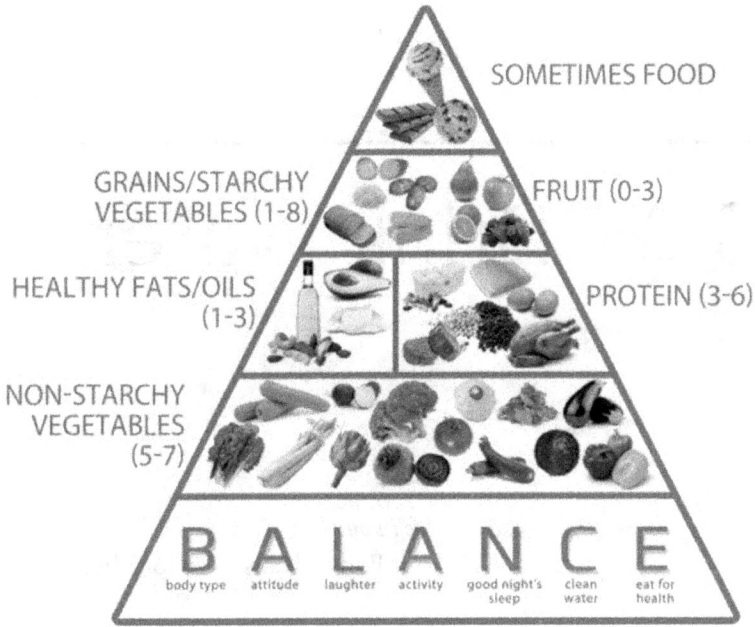

In BALANCE Food Pyramid

Chapter Seven

LEG 2 – Drink Water

"Water is the medium in which life in our body is expressed."
Dr. Batmanghelidj, Your Body's Many Cries for Water

INFORMATION CENTRE

L astly, for this Leg, a quick look at water.

At conception, a baby is surrounded by water, and during its nine months of pre-birth growth, it is carried in a water-filled amniotic sac. And after birth, though we see very little of it, our body fluids are everywhere. Between 57-70% of our body weight is water. That water starts by filling and bathing our body's approximately 37 trillion cells. Then, it makes up the fluid that travels the roughly 62,000 miles of veins and arteries in our body. Ninety-eight percent of intestinal, gastric, saliva, and pancreatic juices are water, and 92% of our blood and tears are water. Water goes virtually everywhere and surrounds almost every bit of tissue in our system.

Water holds nutritive factors in solution and acts as their transportation medium. Another transport function is holding body wastes and toxins in solution and carrying them to where they can be safely removed from the body. Water also acts as a lubricant for our joints and soft tissues. Water provides the liquid necessary for the digestion of food, helps maintain average body temperature, and provides the medium for red blood cells to transport oxygen to the tissues.

Pure water is also one of the best natural protections against various infectious diseases, including influenza, pneumonia, whooping cough, and measles. Your tissues' performance and resistance to injury depend on the quality and quantity of water you drink. When supplied with sufficient pure water, the cells can more easily defend against viral attacks. If body cells are water-starved, they become parched, dry, and shriveled, making them easy prey for viruses.

Drink sufficient clean, slightly alkaline water. Not distilled and not overly alkaline (pH of 8-9 is suitable). Distilled and higher alkaline water can be short-term options, but long-term use can be problematic. With distilled water, one can suffer potential mineral loss, excess acidity, and increased intake of any matter not removed but instead concentrated with distillation. Water that has gone through a multi-step process that includes the removal of both organic contaminants and most chemicals and produces a slight increase in alkalinity (again, that pH of 8-9) is ideal for most people.

How Much Is Enough?

While everyone is different (and will be moving in unique ways, in unique environmental circumstances), drinking roughly .5-1 ounce/water for every pound of body weight (60-120 ounces or 7.5-15 cups for a 120-pound person) is an excellent place to start.

The range is based on factors such as age, climate, exertion, and temperature.

Are you on track with water intake? Simply start by drinking when you are thirsty. There is no need to guzzle water when your body is not giving you "drink now" messages. And note that other beverages, such as herbal teas and juices, help fulfill fluid intake.

Then, use this quick "Am I drinking enough water?" guideline. Other than your morning void, which will be more concentrated and darker colored, or if you are taking certain supplements (B complex, for example, will often produce darker color urine), while urine color will fluctuate throughout the day, it should be relatively light-colored.

REST STOP

Time to take a break and digest information!

Take 10 minutes of calm to Rest with the following questions:

- Do I get enough water?

- Do I need to get a cleaner water source or, at the very least, start with a pitcher-type filtration system?

Next, Stop for 10 minutes of quiet (sitting or slowly walking). Keep your mind as clear and open as possible, and just listen. Jot down any responses that may arise.

ROADWORK

Choose the option that most resonates with you. Note the option and your response in your *Trip Log*.

Option 1 – You knew this was coming. If needed, drink more water! Estimate and then keep track of the amount of water you consume each day for a week. Count water, juice, and clear, non-caffeinated teas as part of your intake. If your intake is low, here are a few suggestions to increase water intake:

- Ensure your water tastes good. At the very least, use a pitcher-type filter to eliminate chlorine and other easily removed contaminants.

- Increase flavor with sliced lemons, limes, or cucumbers.

- Find a selection of herbal teas you enjoy and add them to your daily fluid intake. If the thought of herbal tea makes you gag—too weak, too flavorless—try a rooibos tea. Besides being full of beneficial antioxidants, this South African tea is more hearty-tasting and full-flavored. Even most of my caffeine-loving clients find quality rooibos tea not just tolerable but enjoyable!

- Fill a pitcher with your desired daily water intake. Set it by the sink or refrigerator and drink it throughout the day, finishing it before bed. After you've spent a couple of days chugging ½ the pitcher right at bedtime and had a whack of nighttime bathroom breaks to show for it, you'll likely remember to drink earlier in the day!

Option 2 – Is water intake already "up to speed?" Dig deeper into what's in your grocery cart and look at where sugar in your diet might come from.
- Check out the list of ingredients on any packaged food, noting anything that smacks of sweetness (sugars, dried fruits). Note that ingredients are listed in order of volume, with the highest volume percentage at the top.

- Note, too, that sugar can appear in many forms in the ingredient list: everything from honey, barley malt, molasses, cane syrup, and more to anything with an "ose" ending, such as sucrose, maltose, and glucose.

- Then, for a reality check, review the nutrition panel itself. Note the grams of sugar contained in one serving of the food. Realize that based on guidelines from groups such as the World Health Organization, the recommended daily amount of "free sugar" intake (added sugar plus sugars naturally present in the food) for optimum metabolic wellness and reducing the risk of chronic diseases is 10-25 g/day (or less than 10% of total energy intake).

Where's the Sugar? And How the Heck Do You Know How Much?

Don't necessarily have a clue what, for example, 24 g of sugar even looks like? Not to worry, most of us don't. Instead, divide the grams of sugar by 4 (there are 4.2 g of sugar per teaspoon); in this example, 24/4 = 6.

Now, head to the sugar bowl and count it out. Six teaspoons of sugar. That's six teaspoons of sugar in the tiny box of apple juice or "healthy" granola bar or in ½ of that bottle of energy drink (that no one EVER drinks only ½ of at the time, so you might want to do the visual exercise of measuring out 12 teaspoons of sugar!).

Do the math. Figure out exactly how much sugar you're eating. That's where the rubber meets the road!

TRAVELLER ASSISTANCE – OCC: A Three-Step Action Plan for Healthy Self-Awareness

Talking about what you choose to put in your mouth is a big topic. It is charged with all kinds of memories, emotions, and body|mind|spirit responses (especially, as in my case, when it included examining my sugar intake!). As I discuss with clients, food comes wrapped in much more than cellophane, cardboard, brown paper, and string.

Whenever you take Rest Stops around food (or, for that matter, around any of the other wellness topics that follow), give yourself the grace to put in place the three following steps:

1. **Practice Objectivity.** Be as open as possible to the suggested work or tools by taking a step back and viewing the situation and your responses as if you were a third-party observer. Your behavior will be fueled by something. Dig a bit and see where it takes you.

2. **Practice Curiosity.** Without judgment, note any physical, emotional, or spiritual responses to the suggestions in your *Trip Log*. Ask yourself why you might be having that response. What was I thinking? Where

did those thoughts come from? And what reactions did the thoughts promote?

3. **Practice Compassion.** We typically act in ways that make the most sense to us. The challenge comes when what seemed an excellent choice in the past no longer serves us. Be kind to your younger self. Thank her for her help. Let her know you've got some great new tools that will better support both of you and permit you to let go of the old ways of functioning so that you can embrace the new.

SOUVENIR

Your Leg 2 gift for all the hard work you've put in thus far is to, before you head to bed, give yourself an extra measure of compassion in whatever loving form that takes with you:

- A steaming mug of your favorite hot chocolate.

- A 30-minute date with that novel you've been wanting to finish.

- A leisurely walk around the block in the warm or brisk night air, depending on your location.

- Simply heading to bed early.

Whatever says, in the healthiest way possible, "Thank you for all you do for me; we've got this!" . . . do it.

Chapter Eight

LEG 3 - Body Type for Metabolic Health

SUMMARY – Travel Size Version

Where in This Leg, You Discover Your Metabolic Type and Optimal Fuel Mix!

Diagnostic #2 - Dietary Needs Assessment

First things first! Be sure to download and complete the Dietary Needs Assessment metabolic typing quiz I use with clients. You'll find it here (https ://www.inbalancelm.com/MHR_DNA).

From that, you'll determine whether or not you are a Protein Body Type (parasympathetic dominant, concerning the autonomic nervous system, typically a fast oxidizer/digester of food, and a very efficient fat storer), a Carbohydrate Body Type (sympathetic dominant, concerning the autonomic nervous system, typically a slow oxidizer/digester of food, and not very efficient at storing fat) or a Balanced Body Type that lands somewhere in between a Protein and Carbohydrate Body Type.

Then, we'll unpack what that means for food intake, energy production, and healthy fat stores.

Myth Busting

Though the word "myth" originally meant truth (who knew, eh?), we'll use it here to bust a few food and body fallacies that can trip you up on your way to energy, vitality, and optimal metabolic health!

Myth #1 - The food industry has your best interests at heart.

Myth #2 - Every body needs the same diet.

Macronutrients (AKA Your Fuel Mix)

Here, you'll discover your ideal food choices to support metabolic health best, how they help feed your unique body, and why you might want to load your plate with them in specific percentages.

For history buffs, we'll briefly examine the timeline of eating for humankind and then ensure you understand what foods contain the proteins, fats, and carbohydrates you need to fuel your metabolic type optimally.

Metabolic Typing Basics

Then, for those for whom the concept of Body Typing or Metabolic Typing is new, we will cover a bit of biology. Again, if you're looking for metabolic health, energy, and vitality, we will discuss how body typing guides what should best end up on your plate and in your mouth!

Digging a Little Deeper

You'll also learn more about Faith Goals (dreams) vs. Action Goals (practice) and why knowing and acting on the difference can turn energy—for as long as it takes you to read this book—into energy, health, and vitality for life. You will also understand "clean" food sources, discover four "ask these for the rest of your life" questions . . . oh, and learn a little Japanese!

Chapter Nine

LEG 3 – Discover Your Body Type

"Can't I just get healthy with an eat-everything-in-moderation diet?"

An oft-asked question during a client's first consult

O r this variation: "My brother (or friend or co-worker or neighbor or ____) got healthy (lost weight, cured his ____) on a Keto (or Paleo or vegetarian or flexitarian or vegan or ___) diet. Can't I do what they did and get the same results?"

Or equally common: "I should just do a better job of following the Canada Food Guide (or the US My Plate Guide or any other country's food recommendations), and I'll feel great, right?"

Good questions. And the answer (spoiler alert . . . it's "not likely") is best prefaced with discovering your genetically predisposed body type and some serious myth-busting. Something this Leg is full of!

Diagnostic #2 - Discover Your Body Type

First, however, a recap. Hopefully, one of your biggest takeaways from Leg 2 of your wellness journey is that if you genuinely want to reach your better-health destination, you'll want to concentrate, at least 80% of the time, on eating real food, as close as possible to its original form, and on not falling prey to food fanaticism.

In this Leg, we explore body typing or metabolic typing, the unique way you digest, store, and utilize your food intake. That means that on top of the Three Food Foundations and Five Food Keys, we'll be looking at why it is helpful to personalize your proportions of real food macronutrients (protein, fat, and carbohydrate-rich foods) and how to do that in the most effective (lots of real-life benefits!) and the simplest (no degree in rocket science needed) way.

Be Sure You Have Completed the Dietary Needs Assessment

How do you find out your body type? Before you start, you will need to complete the Dietary Needs Assessment (a metabolic typing survey) included with purchasing this book. It is the assessment I use with my clients, and you get free access:

https://www.inbalancelm.com/MHR_DNA or here.

Completion will take a few minutes, so grab a hot peppermint tea or a cool glass of water and get on the road to discovering information that will serve you well for the rest of your life: your optimal fuel mix! Once you know whether your body does better on a dietary plan with a higher proportion of carbohydrates (on the Dietary Needs Assessment, S or Sx), fats and proteins (on the Dietary Needs Assessment, P or Px), or a balanced intake (on the Dietary Needs Assessment, a B), come on back, I'll introduce you to Jane, and we'll unpack what eating for your metabolic type looks like in real life!

Body Type for Health - Myth Busting

There are lots of ways to say that we're all different; I believe Chris Masterjohn, PhD Nutritional Science, states that fact in one of the best ways possible and gives us a great introduction to the impact of epigenetics on metabolic health:

> *"I do not believe that everyone has the same nutritional needs. I personally do best when I eat a diet rich in animal products. The body, however, has no respect for government guidelines or any person's theory of nutritional superiority; instead, its appetite for nutrition is determined by its molecular and physiological needs at any given moment, on any given day, according to the many factors of the environment, circumstance, and the many biochemical idiosyncrasies of the individual that it must face."*

INFORMATION CENTRE

With a focus on eating according to your body type or genetic responses to different types of macronutrients, you can significantly improve your metabolic health in three primary ways:

1. **Improved nutrient use and metabolic efficiency** – When you eat in a way that is more in line with your specific dietary requirements, you can enhance the way your body processes and utilizes the nutrients. When you get, for example, the higher intake of saturated fat that you require or the lessened intake of carbohydrates that you do better on, your body can operate more efficiently and increase energy levels.

2. **Reduced risk of metabolic disease** – Genetic-based food plans are generally more effective in efficiently regulating blood sugar levels (and fostering appropriate waist size) than one-size-fits-all generic dietary recommendations.

3. **Enhanced personal and psychological well-being** – Trial-and-error wellness approaches (often emphasizing the "error") can lead to frustration and a lack of motivation to pursue wellness practices. A personalized game plan significantly contributes to follow-through and gaining positive benefits. Those improved physical health outcomes can foster better emotional and mental health outcomes.

Finally, when you understand how your body uniquely processes nutrients and adjust your food intake accordingly, you improve metabolic health in general. In addition, your wellness practices are now more aligned with *preventative health measures* geared to your risk factors and needs.

As promised, I have a story about one of my clients, who I will call Jane, to illustrate the value of knowing your body type!

Jane's Story

My new client, Jane, was a lovely older, post-menopausal woman. Unfortunately, her health had been steadily declining over the previous decade, and she now struggled with arthritis, digestive issues, headaches, insomnia, and depression. She had also been consistently increasing in size with the excess body fat she was accumulating, mainly gathering around her abdominal area.

As I reviewed Jane's intake forms with her, I noted that she'd begun eating a vegetarian diet about a dozen years prior. I also noted that on her Dietary Needs Assessment, she'd scored as a Px, needing a higher intake of healthy fat, fewer carbohydrates, and a modest intake of red meat.

I gently asked if there was a specific reason she had switched to a vegetarian diet. Religious reasons, perhaps? Animal rights concerns, maybe?

"Oh no," Jane loudly proclaimed as she sat there in physical and emotional pain that had increased dramatically during the time she'd been vegetarian. Then, looking at me as if I was a slightly daft nutritionist, continued, "It's better for you!"

Understand that this story is not meant to be a "slam" or an insult against my client. Most of us act on reasons that make great sense to us. That's exactly what Jane had done.

Jane's Road Blocks

Unfortunately, until she met me, Jane hadn't understood the Road Blocks of unsound information: not understanding that while a vegetarian diet can be a perfect eating plan for some people, it is a terrible eating plan for others; not knowing that for some people, the gluten in many grains can contribute to inflammation and brain fog; and not realizing that many vegetarian protein sources are also relatively high in carbohydrate content.

Jane's Traffic Jams

Jane also had some unconscious Traffic Jams at play. She'd been raised with a high degree of loyalty to follow through. She'd been taught that once you start something, you finish it. Whether that was a work project, home renovations, or a choice about how to eat best, once you decided, there was no turning back. That meant that rather than considering food as a culprit, her negative body|mind|spirit responses were attributed to stress. Or the weather. Or simply aging.

As we gently unpacked her dietary decisions and I began discussing the benefits of discovering and eating per her ideal fuel mix, Jane became willing to make some small shifts. She eliminated gluten-containing grains for a month. She started eating small amounts of cleanly-sourced wild-caught salmon and free-range eggs. She ditched her "low fat" plan (yup, that had been paired with the vegetarian diet because it too had been touted as "better for you!") and began incorporating increasing amounts of extra virgin olive oil, butter, coconut oil, and avocado into her daily food plan.

Jane's Results

In a matter of days, Jane began to see minor improvements. Her joints moved more easily and with less pain. She was less bloated after meals. And over the next few weeks, positive change continued. Jane's headaches began to appear less frequently and with less severity. She noticed a lightening in her mood and experienced deeper, more restful sleep. Her body began using some of her stored fat for fuel, shifting toward a body size that felt more comfortable.

All that change. Simply by moving from real food to real food in her "optimal fuel mix."

Optimal Fuel Mix

What do I mean by that term? Well, to mix our metaphors (or rather, our body type descriptions), Jane went from treating herself like a regular gas mid-size car to a diesel-run pick-up truck. Once her body began getting the ratio of protein, fat, and carbohydrate-rich fuel on which it was best designed to function, the only way forward was straight down the highway to her ultimate metabolic wellness destination!

Like many of us, Jane fell prey to a couple of common diet myths (no one, least of all me, is pointing fingers here!). Before I help you discover your optimal fuel mix, let's bust those myths to keep you from getting tripped up in an unsound information Road Block (that every body needs the same diet) or completely gridlocked in an unsound thinking Traffic Jam (that the food industry has your best interests at heart).

Let's start with the Traffic Jam.

Myth #1 – The Food Industry Has Your Best Interests at Heart

You would think that if a food item is found in a grocery store—or promoted in a magazine you saw in the grocery store checkout line—it would be good for you. As I've already mentioned, however, there are a lot of items sold or advertised as food that aren't food.

As sad, disheartening, and discouraging as it is, the food industry is not your best friend when it comes to wellness.

MYTH BUSTING

1

**The Food Industry Has Your
Best Interests at Heart**
Food is big business; in
general, the industry is
beholden to profit, boards
and shareholders.

2

**Every Body Needs the
Same Diet**
Instead of focusing on the
"right diet" start exploring
what might be the "right diet
for you!"

Metabolic Health Roadmap Myth Busting

I imagine almost everyone already knows this, but I will repeat it for emphasis: food is big business! Major corporations are competing for your food dollars, and make no mistake: it is a competition. The game includes, among other things, massive amounts of money spent on advertising and the manipulation of our recommended food intake guidelines by industry "experts."

First, let's cut these corporations some slack. Many of the food companies are publicly traded. They are required to work toward maximum profit and are beholden, not to you, but to their shareholders. Simply put, it's not about you; it's just business.

It becomes very unhelpful, however, when an "it's just business" corporation crosses a line and is seen as an expert in the health and wellness of the consumers to whom products are being marketed.

Food Guides – To Follow or Not to Follow?

I've often worked in classroom situations where teachers are doing their best to instill a value for national food guidelines in their students, and in the case of those students' parents, trying to feed their kids, according to Canada's (or other countries') governmental food guide recommendations.

Did you know that before releasing a new food guide in 2019, when Canada's Food Rainbow was last revised, 4 of the 12-panel members—25% of that committee—were employed in the food industry by corporations that would be significantly affected by the Guide's recommendations?

Several of those, for example, were the nutrition education manager for the BC Dairy Foundation, executive director of the Vegetable Oil Industry of Canada, and director of scientific and regulatory affairs at the Food & Consumer Products Manufacturers of Canada—the latter represented the interests of corporations such as PepsiCo, Frito-Lay, and Coca-Cola.

I'll let you decide how much final say you think those members had on that food guide version. The fact the committee recommended every single Canadian have between 2-4 daily servings of dairy, consume 2-3 tablespoons of unsaturated fat (read vegetable oil) every day, and only "limit" their consumption of trans-fats, a fat found in many processed snack foods, (when we knew, even at that time, that there is, in fact, no safe amount of trans fat consumption) and I think you'll have some idea!

In 2016, experts (actual experts such as dieticians and health care practitioners), speaking to the Canadian Standing Senate Committee on Obesity, summed things up nicely: "Food guides, although they may vary from country to country, too often reflect the financial interests of the dominant food businesses."

They went even further when they said that, at best, the Canada Food Guide had done nothing to alleviate obesity rates in Canada and, at worst, had contributed to our increasing overweight and obese population.

Canada's current food guide makes better recommendations. Still, it has a way to go with the relatively large amount of fruit and other carbohydrates recommended and a lack of sound guidance on healthy fat intake. Unfortunately, it still advocates a one-size-fits-all approach.

Myth #2 – Every Body Needs the Same Diet

For several years, I taught nutrition to teens and young adults through a non-profit that supported new immigrants to Canada. It was one of my favorite nutrition gigs!

Picture a roomful of young people, originally from all over the world, coming together to learn how to eat "right" in their new country. And having the absolute best questions during discussion time—"Why do you have so many kinds of milk?", "What's with the watery skim variety?" and "Why is the chicken in the store such a funny color?"!

Three Food Foundations Revisited

After giving them the Three Food Foundations (the ones you just got!) I asked them where they were from and how their family had eaten before they'd arrived in Canada. I also asked about their grandparents' history with food. Then, I suggested that the class participants keep eating as close as possible to the way they had been raised, except in situations where they had immigrated from bigger cities and had, perhaps, already begun adopting more ultra-processed food intake or from countries experiencing war or drought or other challenges that negatively impacted food security and a healthy food supply.

How Did YOUR Great-Grandparents Eat?

Don't start now if you didn't previously drink milk or eat dairy. If your family historically ate a lot of rice and little bread, don't get on the wheat train. If legumes were your main protein source, avoid a carnivore diet. If you generally eat regular dairy, avoid the low-fat variety. You need at least some fat in your dairy product to help process the calcium in it, and if it's low-fat, it generally has added sugar to make up for the fact that flavourful fat has been removed.

Eat For Who YOU Are

While a deep dive into the specific genes that impact how we metabolize and utilize food is beyond the scope of the *Metabolic Health Roadmap*, it is helpful to understand that the Dietary Needs Assessment gives genetic clues.

As a reminder, genes act as a set of directions that build a person's features (traits) and provide the information cells need to differentiate, reproduce, and grow. Not all single nucleotide polymorphisms (SNPs)—genetic variations—affect health, but some impact wellness outcomes and can affect how we respond to protein, fat, and carbohydrates. SNPs can also play a role in our responses to stress.

Along with considering the dietary patterns of our family of origin, discovering body type (a bird's-eye view of the way the body metabolizes food and the part of the Autonomic Nervous System that is more dominant) is another excellent tool for avoiding "same diet for all" recommendations.

Whether you are an S or Sx Body Type (have the genetic makeup to tolerate a higher percentage of carbohydrates in your fuel mix and often need less fat and protein), a P or Px Body Type (have the genetic makeup that generally requires a higher percentage of fat and protein—including some animal protein—and less carbohydrates in your fuel mix) or a B Body Type (have the genetic makeup that generally needs a balanced ratio), for the rest of the book, I'd encourage you to set aside thoughts of the "right diet" and instead focus on the "right food plan for YOU"!

You may have a Road Block or two to detour around and a couple of Traffic Jams to dissolve, but once you do so, you'll have made room for a lot of open highway on your way to optimal metabolic wellness!

REST STOP

Time to take a break and digest information!

Take 10 minutes of calm to Rest with the following questions:

1. Where have I been tripped up by food industry advertising or the belief that there is one correct diet?

2. Are those obstacles Road Blocks (unsound information that, now that it is corrected, should be easy to work around) or Traffic Jams (unsound thinking about, for example, my "deserving" of sugar or my belief that my family's "fat genes" make it impossible to reach a comfortable-for-me size)?

Next, Stop for 10 minutes of quiet (sitting or slowly walking). Keep your mind as clear and open as possible, and just listen. Jot down any responses that may arise.

ROADWORK

Choose the option that most resonates with you. Note the option and your response in your *Trip Log*.

Option 1 – Take a look at a magazine (physical or digital) that contains food advertising. How many of the advertisements include words like "healthy," "natural," or "good for you"? Are those words being used to describe what you now consider real food, as close as possible to its original form? Or are they more likely attempts at "greenwashing" and trying to make foods appear more sustainably or environmentally grown or healthier for us than they are?

Based on the magazine's photos, how much inference is there that eating or serving a particular product will produce positive results such as fitness, happiness, a new relationship, or winning a host/hostess of the year award?

Option 2 – Look at a magazine (physical or digital) and think about your body shape and size relative to what you see pictured in the magazine's articles and advertising. Do you have what is portrayed as an "ideal" body shape and size? Does that matter to you? Do you understand the philosophies, ad spend (marketing budget), and latest trends that go into "idealized" bodies?

What would you like your shape and size to be at the end of your wellness destination (your vision or Faith Goal)? Is this based on health and wellness or societal ideology?

Dig into why you believe what you do about your body. Where can you begin to shift Traffic Jams (unsound thinking)?

The Fallacy (and False Allure) of "Ideal" Bodies

Keep in mind that specific body shapes will seem more highly regarded than others depending on the current fashion cycle, healthful accuracy of the latest food trends, and degree of social influence. This is another book's worth of material, but for now, recognize that much of what we value in fashion and beauty is shaped by dominant cultural thinking, which is not always good! Notice if that "unsound thinking" Traffic Jam influences your beliefs about your body or determines what you picture your body looking like in your Faith Goal.

Recognize, too, that S and Sx bodies are typically leaner and often, but not always, taller. P and Px bodies generally are larger, rounder, and often, but not always, shorter. Those are not mistakes. They are a genetic design feature.

Each size and shape has had its on-again/off-again run at being most prized and the height of fashion and desire. Think extra fat stores helping with survival or the lovingly—and sometimes lustfully—described term "Rubenesque."

Whatever your genetically predisposed body type, remember that one is not better than the other; it is only different and equally to be valued.

TRAVELLER ASSISTANCE – Faith Goals vs. Action Goals

For consistent forward movement, we need two types of goals: Faith (or dream or vision) Goals and Action Goals (steps we put into actual practice). Faith Goals are big-picture in nature. They are the destinations of our wellness journey.

My Faith Goals included things like:

- Sleeping through the night.

- Having a yawn-free afternoon.

- Reaching a more comfortable-for-me waist circumference.

- Having enough energy and clarity to smoke my husband at racquetball!

However, to get from where we are to that Faith Goal, we need clear, actionable, and measurable steps (Action Goals). Otherwise, a Faith Goal is merely a pipe dream that will never achieve fruition.

Reaching That Goal!

In the words of Keith J. Cunningham in his excellent and highly recommended book, *The Road Less Stupid:*

"The primary reason most goals are never achieved ... is because they are hollow, generalized statements of hope and not rigorous nonnegotiable standards, plans, and measurable drivers."

So, along with my Faith Goals, I also had Action Goals that were scheduled, trackable, No Matter Whats (more on NMWs later) and included things like:

- Take 2 mg of melatonin 15 minutes before bedtime.

- Practice racquetball at the gym across from my office during two lunch breaks a week; invite my co-worker Viviane to join me.

- Only go into the staff room for herbal tea or to eat the cleanly sourced and packed lunch I'd brought, and walk on the opposite side of the room as the honor snack box location!

Dream big, come up with a wellness big picture "Why" that scares the heck out of you and a destination that is full of hope. Then, fill in your journey itinerary with Action Goals that you can easily measure and quickly follow. We know that Action Goals cannot require the uncertain cooperation of our bodies or someone else. Thus, even though I would invite Viviane, my co-worker, to practice racquetball with me, I would not make my hitting the court dependent on whether or not she was available that day.

Be sure Action Goals are trackable, sustainable, and attainable by you and you alone. That includes ensuring goals are not dependent upon the "uncertain cooperation of your body"! If you're not sure what I mean by that, read on! Most of my clients don't initially get it either because we aren't taught this vital truth in goal setting.

Why I Don't Recommend Weight Loss as an Action Goal

As a Faith Goal, I wanted to get my waist circumference closer to ½ of my height. As it was, it didn't feel like a comfortable shape for my body, and it was extra abdominal/visceral fat, which was not a super healthy type of body fat to carry.

I could not, however, control how quickly my body would shed that excess stored fat (nor could anyone else, for that matter). That means that a weight release goal requires the uncertain cooperation of my body. I don't know its "to-do" list and am uncertain whether its timeline will cooperate with my goals. Maybe it is cleaning plaque from my arteries, repairing a slight ankle sprain, or creating new bone. All things my body—while doing an excellent job of keeping me alive and well—has prioritized over moving me down a pant size or two.

I did, however, control the foods I put in my mouth, the number of steps I took in a day, how I thought of and spoke about my body, the time I turned my light off at night, and whether I'd listed three things for which I was grateful before that light went off. Viewing goals this way may seem like an insignificant difference or mere semantics. Think, however, how you would feel at the end of a week knowing that while your Faith Goal of being a particular body size/shape/fitness level had yet to be achieved, you had accomplished every one of the Action Goals you had set for yourself.

Which feels more compassionate?

- Feeling discouraged and disappointed that the dreams had yet to materialize.

- Being grateful and proud that you followed through on the small action steps you said were important to you.

Note, too, that if you've created relevant and proven Action Goals to support your Faith Goals, completing them makes it much more likely that your Faith Goals will eventually be reached!

As an aside, note that not only did I have a Faith Goal to beat my 6'2", double-my-size, super athletic husband at racquetball, but I also wanted to play competitively.

By taking consistent action, I was soon regularly beating Mark (much to his chagrin), and my doubles partner, Viviane, and I went on to play women's doubles at the top Canadian level under Pro. The lesson was noted, and I'll reiterate it here. The more I consistently followed through on my Action Goals, the more I increased my likelihood of realizing my Faith Goals!

Oh, and one more aside? The excess abdominal fat eventually melted away, too! In my body's timing and order of health priority.

FAITH GOALS VS. ACTION GOALS

Knowing and acting on the difference goes a long way to more easily reaching your wellness destination!

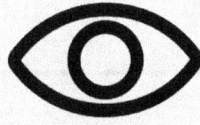

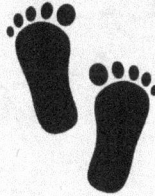

Faith Goals

Faith or dream goals are big picture and vision. They require a measure of faith to believe you can be, do, have and give what you see!

Action Goals

Action goals are specific and measurable. They should not require the uncertain cooperation of your body or anyone else.

Faith Goals vs. Action Goals

Chapter Ten

LEG 3 - Body Type: Getting Started

"Food, in the end, in our own tradition, is something holy. It's not about nutrients and calories. It's about sharing. It's about honesty. It's about identity."

Louise Fresco, Dutch scientist and writer known for her work on globally sustainable food production

INFORMATION CENTRE

If you've completed the Dietary Needs Assessment (DNA) linked to in this Leg's introductory section, you'll now know if you are an S (Sympathetic Dominant; typically do better on a dietary plan that includes a higher percentage of healthy carbohydrate-rich food and a lower percentage of healthy fats); an Sx (Sympathetic Dominant Extreme; an S to the max!); a P (Parasympathetic Dominant; typically do better on a dietary plan that includes a higher percentage of healthy fats, a moderate protein intake that includes animal protein, and a much lower percentage of carbohydrate-rich food); a Px (Parasympathetic Dominant Extreme; think a P on steroids!); or a B (Balanced Body Type that does best, generally, on about an equal mix of all three macronutrients).

Now is the time, therefore, to examine the three macronutrients—the building blocks—of your dietary plan: protein, carbohydrates, and fats. But you may have also noticed that, in the previous sections, I mentioned what could be a new-to-you phrase: cleanly-sourced foods. So, let's start there. What do I mean by clean or, as they are sometimes called, "healthy" food sources?

Clean Food Sources

Think back to the "as close as possible to their original form" Food Foundation. That means spending your food dollars on wild-caught rather than farmed fish. That means beef that comes from pasture-raised animals. Free-range chicken and eggs. Olive oil that is pressed the way it has been for generations (choose cold-pressed, extra virgin, or virgin olive oil). Butter rather than margarine ... and on and on.

Another way of looking at clean/healthy sources is to consider the History of Eating. Since we've only recently begun to eat more ultra-processed and less clean foods, we should focus on eating foods with a long history of use.

History of Eating

According to nutrition experts like Jonny Bowden and Jonathan Bailor, if you look at the period that the modern form of humans has existed and consider those tens of thousands of years as just 24 hours, up until 3 minutes ago—11:57 pm—in those almost 24 hours, we stayed healthy and fit eating only what could be hunted, gathered, fished or plucked.

Three minutes ago, people started farming and eating more starch and small amounts of sweets.

People began eating ultra-processed starches and sweets only three seconds ago—at 11:59:57 pm.

And only one second ago—at 11:59:59 pm—people started getting most of their calories from manufactured starch and sweetener-based foodish products.

I'm not just relating this information to those who love learning about the olden days! The history lesson becomes a Traveler Assistance lifesaver for everyone the next time someone tries to disparage your food plan—where you focus on lots of healthy fat, moderate amounts of healthy protein, and modest amounts of safer starches—by describing it as a "fad" diet.

Diets that consist primarily of refined and processed grains and sugars are faddish, particularly when you consider that for at least 99.8% of our history, a diet containing ultra-processed foods—indeed, most government-recommended diet guidelines today—was not even possible!

So, what is possible today? What are your fuel options?

While we require many types of nutrients for optimal health, including mi-cro-nutrients like vitamins and minerals, three primary types of nutrients need to be in pretty much everyone's dietary intake: protein, carbohydrates, and fat.

Two of those three macronutrients have components that are required for life and that the body cannot make: protein (essential amino acids, the building blocks of protein) and fats (essential fatty acids, omega-3s, and omega-6s).

Carbohydrate intake is not critical for life, per se, as our bodies can make carbo-hydrates out of components found in protein and fats. That said, carbohydrates are a vital food source. I recommend that all my clients, regardless of body type, have regular, personalized-for-them carbohydrate intake, especially in vegetable and fruit form, as they contain various other vital nutrients.

Finally, having a ready supply of carbohydrates means our body doesn't have to regularly default to the less efficient and more stress-inducing backup mecha-nisms of supplying energy primarily from fat (ketosis) or protein (gluconeogen-esis).

When looking at proteins and fats, realize, too, that many foods we consider to fall in those categories—legumes for protein, for example, or cheese for fat—also contain a hefty proportion of carbohydrates. So, when I mention a protein-rich food or a fat-rich food, let that be a reminder to reach for foods that have a high percentage of protein or fat in them, not simply something often considered a protein or fat that contains lower levels of that macronutrient and lots of carbohydrate content, as well.

Protein (3-6 servings of protein-rich food a day)

Next to water, protein is the most abundant nutrient in our bodies. We require protein to:

- Develop and maintain muscle, bone, vital organs, blood, hair, nails, and other body tissue.

- Produce hormones, enzymes, antibodies, and blood cells.

- Develop a healthy immune system.

- Fight infection.

- Recover from illness when it strikes.

During digestion, protein is broken down into protein building blocks called amino acids. Our bodies can make eleven of the twenty amino acids commonly recognized in the genetic code we use to form and repair various organs and tissues. The human body cannot synthesize the other nine amino acids, which are regarded as essential as they need to be supplied through diet. Consuming a variety of protein-rich foods is crucial for health maintenance.

Foods that are included in the protein-rich group include:

- Meat (beef, bison, lamb, pork, elk, venison, moose, rabbit).

- Seafood (sardines, trout, anchovies, bluefish, flounder, halibut, Pacific cod, prawns, scallops, sole, wild salmon).

- Poultry (chicken, turkey, Cornish game hen, duck, goose).

- Nuts (almonds, cashews, filberts, pecans, walnuts, pine nuts, Brazil nuts, macadamia nuts, nut butter).

- Seeds (flax, sesame, hemp, sunflower, chia, pumpkin, seed butter).

- Dairy products (cheese, yogurt, kefir, cottage cheese, milk).

- Eggs (chicken, duck, goose, quail).

- Legumes (split peas, snap peas, snow peas, chickpeas, peanuts, lentils, and beans–pinto, Romano, black, white, kidney), though they contain a fair amount of carbohydrates, as well.

Protein Body Types (P & Px): require a higher percentage of protein-rich foods in their daily fuel mix. For optimum mood or physical and mental energy, they usually need to include, regularly, at least small amounts of what is called the medium or higher purine-rich proteins found in red meats, darker poultry (game birds or thighs and drumsticks of chicken and turkey), wild game, organ meats, and richer seafood such as anchovies, sardines, herring, and salmon. Purines are a common chemical compound—both found in foods and produced naturally by the body—that, for some body types, need to be kept in moderation as they can lead to elevated levels of uric acid (which can, in turn, result in gout).

Carbohydrate Body Types (S & Sx): require less protein-rich food in their daily fuel mix and usually need more of it in a lower purine-rich form, such as eggs, cold-water fish, legumes, nuts and seeds, and fruits. They often see a negative impact on mood, energy, mental clarity, or physical health (inflammation, gout) with higher purine-rich foods.

Balanced Body Types (B): usually do best with a regular and moderate protein intake, combining higher and lower purine-rich foods. They must experiment with the exact fuel mix to see what most suits their body type.

Fats (1-3 servings a day)

Among other functions, fats are used by the body to create cell membranes, help with inflammation and pain, grow healthy hair, skin, and nails, and work to produce and balance hormones. There are healthy fats, some of which are essential (the body cannot make; need to be supplied through diet), unhealthy fats that should, generally, be avoided, and saturated fat, a healthy fat we can handle in varying genetically determined amounts.

Healthy Fats

Nuts, seeds, avocados, and oils such as extra virgin olive oil, virgin olive oil, coconut oil, butter, tallow, sesame oil, grapeseed oil, walnut oil, sunflower oil, hemp oil, and flaxseed oil supply healthy fats. Healthy fats are also found in oily fish—such as salmon, halibut, herring, cod, sardines, and mackerel—dairy products, marbled meat, and the skin of fish and poultry.

Monounsaturated Fats (MUFAs) found in foods such as olive and avocados or olive and avocado oil are widely recognized as beneficial, especially for insulin sensitivity and cardiovascular health. They should play a moderate role in most people's diets and can be consumed daily.

Saturated fats have ridden the in-vogue/out-of-vogue or good fat/bad fat roller coaster for decades. In fact, a daily intake of saturated fat is essential to support many body functions, including cell membrane integrity and healthy hormone production—saturated fats play a role in synthesizing hormones like estrogen and testosterone.

Saturated fats should be consumed in moderation (genetic factors indicate a range of 22-40 g/day) but have a well-earned and traditional place in a balanced diet. Suppose you are not sure of your metabolic requirement. In that case, keeping to an average amount of about 28 g/day can be helpful until you determine (through, for example, genetic testing) your exact bio-individual needs.

Essential Fatty Acids (EFAs), with that "essential" term again, means your body can't make this nutrient, and you must get it through your diet. Essential Fatty Acids (EFAs) are fats as necessary as vitamins and minerals for optimum health and must be supplied daily through diet or supplements.

Unlike other healthy fats prominent in energy production, EFAs are used mainly for hormonal, structural, and nerve functions. They are found primarily in oily fish and some nuts and seeds. We need both a small intake of linoleic acid (LA), an omega-6 fatty acid found in safflower oil, sunflower oil, poppy seeds, hemp seeds, sesame seeds, and wheat germ, as well as alpha-linolenic acid (ALA), an omega-3 fatty acid found in fish and fish oils, flaxseeds, pumpkin seeds, chia seeds, kiwi and walnuts.

Polyunsaturated fatty acids (PUFAs) include omega-3 and omega-6 fatty acids. PUFAs generally have a reputation for being health-promoting. However, there is concern that high ratios of omega-6 to omega-3 fatty acids, in particular, can contribute to conditions such as chronic inflammation, energy production dysregulation, and fat storage.

Found in most nut and seed oils and often used in producing processed foods, many individuals get too high an intake of PUFAs. That volume and the poor quality of much of that intake (heated, bleached, deodorized) can contribute to adverse health effects. Keep polyunsaturated fat intake low-moderate, and as much as possible, have it as natural and quality-processed as possible.

Saturated and monounsaturated fats have specific physiological roles important in metabolic health. Key to healthy fat intake, therefore, is source and ratios. Optimize your balance, set it on the foundation of your Food Foundations and Food Keys, and you'll enhance hormone balance, support cellular function, and improve your overall metabolic health.

Cooking With Oils

Most nut and seed oils should not be heated as cooking destroys the essential fatty acids or encourages rancidity.

Coconut oil, a long-used saturated fat, is an exception to the "no heat" rule and, for those who can handle higher saturated fat intake (generally P, Px types), is an excellent choice for cooking, notably higher heat cooking. Coconut oil also works well for sautéing foods or baking, although butter and olive oil can also be used at low-moderate heat. For butter and olive oil, start with a cold pan, add the fat, and slowly heat the pan. Less heat-resistant oils (extra virgin olive oil, walnut oil) should not be used for cooking but be drizzled on cooked vegetables or used in salad dressings.

Unhealthy Fats

Altered fats—fats that have been negatively impacted by heating or hydrogenation—or fats found in meats with an unhealthy ratio of omega-6 to omega-3 fat fall into the category of unhealthy fats. The higher ratio of omega-6 to omega-3 fat results when animals are fed an abundance of grains rather than grass-fed; it is a ratio that has been linked to inflammation and various chronic diseases.

Realize that even good EFAs can become harmful if heated or altered. Watch both the type of oil you are purchasing and how it is processed (look for as natural, unrefined, and cold-pressed a source as possible). Store oils in dark containers, away from heat and light.

Carbohydrates (number of servings varies by type of carb and body type)

Along with protein and fat, carbohydrates are one of the three macronutrients our bodies use for optimum health. In my food plan recommendations, the carbohydrate-rich food group is divided into three subcategories: grains and starchy vegetables, non-starchy vegetables, and fruit. Because they are derived from plant sources, good-quality carbohydrate-rich foods are usually naturally low in fat and cholesterol. However, once carbohydrate foodstuffs are processed, many of their valuable nutrients are removed or destroyed.

While everyone can benefit from an intake of carbohydrate-rich foods, depending upon body type, the type and amount of carbohydrates eaten daily needs to be monitored. Every body type needs carbohydrates from vegetables, but Protein (P, Px), Carbohydrate (S, Sx), and Balanced (B) Body Types need starchy vegetables, grains, and fruit-source carbohydrates in differing types and amounts.

To achieve optimal wellness, Protein Body Types often need to limit their starchy vegetable intake to 1-2 servings/day, keep their fruit intake to 0-2 servings/day, and strictly limit or avoid grains. Carbohydrate Body Types typically do better on a higher percentage of starchy vegetables, grains, and fruit. Balanced Body Types will need an amount that falls somewhere between the amount that keeps a Protein and Carbohydrate Body Type functioning optimally.

Vegetables (5-10 servings a day)

To help provide the vitamins, minerals, fiber, and enzymes needed to maintain optimal health, most people should eat a minimum of five servings of lower-glycemic vegetables—non-starchy varieties with a slower digestion and absorption rate. If oxalates, a naturally occurring compound found in higher amounts in beans, beer, chocolate, coffee, soy, and some vegetables, are an issue, check high-oxalate food lists and avoid potentially problematic foods such as potatoes, beets and some dark green vegetables like spinach.

Protein Body Types can include high-purine vegetables such as asparagus, spinach, cauliflower, and mushrooms. Carbohydrate Body Types should include more low-purine vegetables such as cabbage, squash, red bell pepper, and beetroot.

Vegetables are versatile and flavourful and can be served in various ways, including in recipes that, believe it or not, can become absolute favorites.

Grains and Starchy Vegetables (1-8 servings a day)

Minimize or eliminate white flour-based products when grains are in your optimal fuel mix. Realize that people have varying tolerances to even natural whole grains. For some, it is an issue with gluten—the protein in many grains, mainly barley, rye, triticale, spelt, bulgur, and wheat.

For others, it may be because of the grain's anti-nutrient components (phytic acid, tannins, saponins, protease inhibitors). Also found in other food crops, such as legumes and some vegetables, these anti-nutrients interfere with processes like digestion and mineral absorption. In these instances, it can be best to use non-gluten grains (quinoa, millet, rice) and starchy vegetables (yams, sweet potatoes, white/red potatoes, taro, plantain, beets) as primary carbohydrate-rich food sources. In addition, to reduce phytic acid—a substance found in many plant-based foods that can bind to minerals such as iron, zinc, and calcium and impair their absorption—and increase nutritional content and digestibility, ensure that grains are sprouted or fermented before serving (sprouted grain bread, f ermented oats).

Fruit (0-3 servings/day)

Fruit is a source of vitamins, minerals, antioxidants, and fiber. While fruit can make an excellent snack, particularly for Carbohydrate and Balanced Body Types, or when paired with nutrient-dense protein-rich food such as nuts or a piece of cheese, it is crucial to monitor the amount of fruit intake for Protein Body Types. Most fruits are high in natural sugars and are best used sparingly and often seasonally by Protein Body Types, those who genetically have less effective carb-response genes, and all body types during a dietary candida-type cleanse.

Fruit juices can play a small part in a healthy diet for some body types (typically Carbohydrate and Balanced Body Types). Generally, however, if you are thirsty, make water your beverage of choice and ensure most of your fruit servings are a whole piece of fruit rather than fruit juice. Hence, you enjoy the additional fiber and nutrient benefits.

How Much is Enough?

And how much should you eat based on the number of servings that suit your type? Until comfortably full and satisfied rather than stuffed or overstuffed. If overeating has been an issue, aim for that helpful 80/20 key, which is about 80% full. Listen to your body and then learn to trust your body as you better determine your satiety levels.

One More Body Type Story . . . This One is Closer to Home!

If you're still wrestling with the concept of an individualized diet, here is one last story for this Leg.

My husband is a Px; after 25 years of doing 100s of these assessments with clients, he is still pretty much the highest number I've seen in that type. I joke with him that while the rest of his body and brain have evolved well into the 21st century, he has yet to move beyond a Neanderthal gut. It thinks his food supply still consists primarily of what he can hunt, fish, pluck, and gather: eggs, roots, bugs, birds, fish, and the occasional dinosaur (that is, then, all parts—including every organ and bit of fat and marrow—gorged on for three weeks straight).

Before I discovered body typing, our family ate a healthy vegetarian diet for over a year.

Mark was slowly getting more and more lethargic (a more challenging time getting to soccer, basketball, and bike riding, and a much easier time getting to the couch to watch those sports); more and more cranky (no longer quickly being pastoral with those closest to him: me and our five kids), and had put on 25 pounds of excess body fat.

After having him complete a brand-new-concept-to-me metabolic typing survey (like the Dietary Needs Assessment you completed) and seeing his scores, our vegetarian-for-everyone-in-the-family days were over.

Once we began incorporating cleanly sourced red meat into our diet plan and upped the healthy fat content (and decreased Mark's carbohydrate intake), in six weeks, I had my energetic, even-tempered, mentally clear husband back. And, yes, he'd also dropped the 25 pounds of excess body fat.

It indeed was a "eureka" moment for me. I realized, loud and clear, that my husband—and everyone else I've ever had the privilege of working with or teaching since—does much better when they eat according to their gut and genetically predisposed body type than according to the, in science and nutrition researcher, Sally Fallon's words, *"politically correct nutrition and the diet dictocrats."*

Finally, look for these secondary benefits when eating right for your type:

- **Energy:** awareness of advertising, Bliss Points, product placement in grocery stores, and convenience.

- **Mental clarity:** recognizing comfort foods, one-size-diet-fits-all beliefs, and equating foods with reward.

- **Balanced moods:** growing in healthier shopping, cooking skills, and ingredient awareness.

- **Comfortable-for-you body size:** developing a "what brings me joy" list, appreciation for YOUR body.

REST STOP

Time to take a break and digest information!

Take 10 minutes of calm to Rest with the following questions:

- Consider any "quick dietary fixes" you may have tried. What led you to give them a try? What were the results?

- Are those obstacles Road Blocks (unsound information that, now that it has been corrected, should be easy to work around) or Traffic Jams (unsound thinking)?

Next, Stop for 10 minutes of quiet (sitting or slowly walking). Keep your mind as clear and open as possible, and just listen. Jot down any responses that may arise.

ROADWORK

Choose the option that most resonates with you. Note the option and your response in your *Trip Log*.

Option 1 – Take a look at the following three Plate Portioning Guides and see if you can begin to eat more closely in alignment with your optimal fuel mix, Protein [Parasympathetic (P) or Parasympathetic Extreme (Px)], Carbohydrate [Sympathetic (S) or Sympathetic Extreme (Sx)], or Balanced (B).

Note the Plate Portioning guides are a "guide" and a beginning point. As you continue through the Legs, I will give additional information and suggestions so you know how to adjust and fine-tune food intake. This, however, is a GREAT starting place!

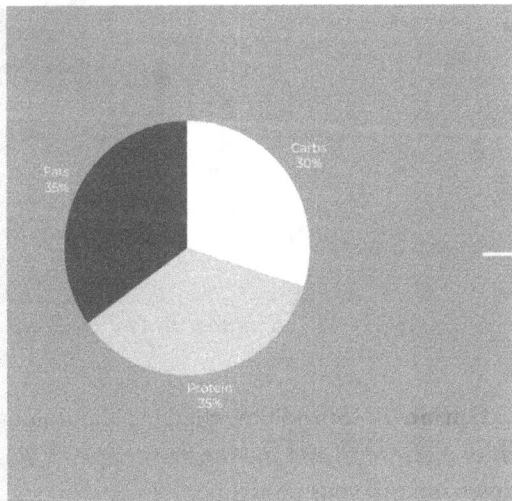

PLATE PORTIONING BY TYPE

PROTEIN BODY TYPE

Genetically designed to conserve energy with the greatest efficiency, P and Px types have the slowest metabolic rates and are most efficient at converting food into stored fat as their energy reserves.

They generally do well to include 30-40% animal protein (including red meat, darker poultry), 30-50% mono and polyunsaturated fats (olive and avocado oils) and saturated fat (butter, lard, coconut oil, animal skin).

This body type has the lowest tolerance for carbohydrates (10-30%); intake of even moderately starchy foods may foster fat storage.

Carbs 30%
Fats 35%
Protein 35%

Protein Body Type Plate Portioning

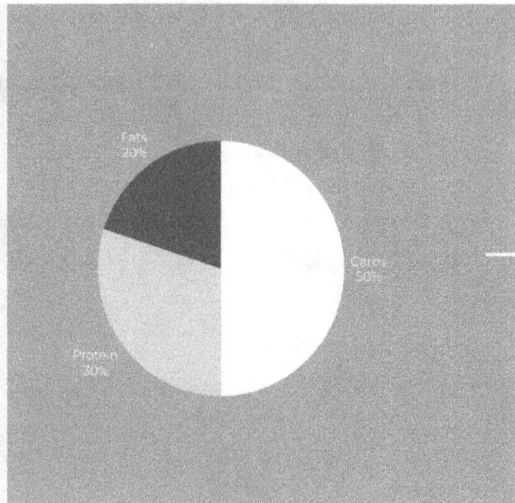

PLATE PORTIONING BY TYPE

CARBOHYDRATE BODY TYPE

Types S and Sx have comparatively fast metabolic rates (energy expenditure), and digestion that is least efficient at converting food into stored fat for energy reserves.

They do best on 30-40% vegetable protein and lighter forms of animal protein (fish, eggs, chicken breast), and on 10-20% monounsaturated or polyunsaturated oils (avocado, olive) rather than on saturated forms of fat (butter, lard, coconut oil).

They typically do well on 40-50% carbohydrates but those, as with any body type's carbs, should be unrefined and low-moderate starch.

Fats 20%

Carbs 50%

Protein 30%

Carbohydrate Body Type Plate Portioning

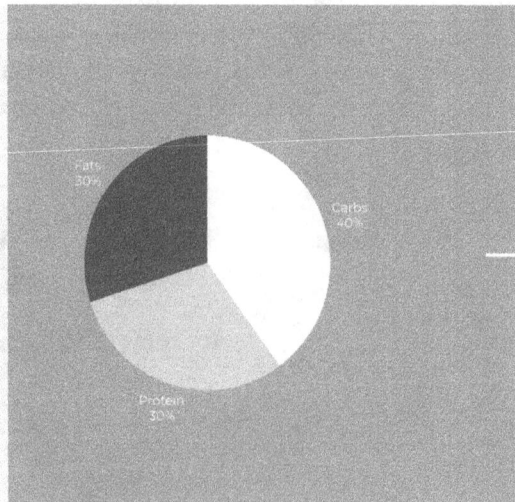

PLATE PORTIONING BY TYPE

BALANCED BODY TYPE

Balanced body types generally have more equal access to both the parasympathetic (P) and sympathetic (S) sides of the autonomic nervous system.

They are balanced metabolizers and do well with a diet blended a little more evenly from all three macronutrients: fat, protein and carbohydrates.

A ratio of 30-40% protein, 35-40% carbohydrates and 20-30% fat is a great place to start.

Fats 30%

Carbs 40%

Protein 30%

Balanced Body Type Plate Portioning

Option 2 – Spend time thinking about how you would describe each of the three macronutrients and the first couple of words that come to your mind. Jot down some of your thoughts.

Now, spend time being curious about where those thoughts and feelings have come from. It's always exciting and often enlightening to discover the misinformation (Road Blocks) and biases or paradigms (Traffic Jams) behind our actions, especially regarding food.

Remember, too, that as you process your responses to these food components, along with objectivity and curiosity, include ample compassion. Generally, we developed thoughts and behaviors that made the most sense to us when they began to occur. Always be kind to that younger version of yourself who did the best they could with the information and experiences they'd had.

Realize that the paradigms and biases (or thoughts and beliefs) that served us (perhaps even kept us alive) in the past may be the very things that keep us "Road Blocked" now. It takes courage to let "Traffic Jam" thoughts go and embrace a new way of thinking.

TRAVELLER ASSISTANCE – 80/20 Rule

There is a Japanese practice called *Hara hachi bu*. In short, it means, "Eat until you're 80% full." Originating in Okinawa, it is a helpful method of thinking about how much you eat and noting when enough is enough. It keeps you from eating rapidly and from overeating when your digestive system has not yet had a chance to register fullness, and it can make you more aware of the tastes, textures, and enjoyment of your food.

Concentrating on the meal (and good conversation), turning off the TV, and putting phones and other devices away makes the practice easier. Using smaller plates and bowls and learning to listen to your body's "almost full" messages can also help grow this skill set.

Note, too, that the 80/20 Rule doesn't just apply to being comfortably full at meal and snack time. You can apply it to a variety of wellness "best practices," including:

- Sleep patterns (hitting your target bedtime and rising time at least 80% of the time)

- Getting enough veggies in a day (at least 80% of the time, eating the optimal type and amount for your body type)

- Sometimes Food guidelines (keeping celebratory foods and drink to no more than 20% of your dietary intake)

No matter the scenario, aiming for 80% will usually get you well on the road to your optimal wellness destination.

Chapter Eleven

LEG 3 - Body Type Basics

"Jack Sprat could eat no fat, His wife could eat no lean; And so betwixt them both, They lick'd the platter clean."

English Nursery Rhyme

INFORMATION CENTRE

Once you have minimized or eliminated the sugar and refined flours and applied all of the other tips I've been recommending over the past few Legs, discovering and then eating and living by your genetically determined metabolic type is the fastest, most effective way to become fit, energetic and mentally sharp that I know (and I've taken a good look at most of them). It's one of the primary factors that sets my wellness methods apart from other coaching programs. It makes what I recommend simple, doable, and effective!

Body Typing: Not the New Kid on the Block

Now, as you'll know from my illustrations over the past few chapters, I didn't invent body typing (or my husband would not have been doing happy dances in the kitchen, celebrating the fact that I'd quit serving him soy grit casseroles and that we were headed out to buy a ¼ of grass-fed beef!).

Metabolic typing has been practiced and studied, in some form or other, for 1000s and 1000s of years. Using assessment tools to interpret tongue symptomatology, pulse, and cold or hot patterns, Traditional Chinese Medicine practitioners "prescribe" a bio-chemically unique course of treatment—herbs, acupuncture, tinctures—and food therapy for each patient.

India's Ayurvedic medicine, elements of which have been practised for 5000 years, also evaluates individuals by constitution or state of body balance. Primary treatment recommendations address one's "dosha" or metabolic type before they address the disease.

Much of modern-day research on body typing has come about as researchers or practitioners were frustrated because some of their clients/patients were getting well on specific dietary and supplement protocols, and other patients/clients, often exhibiting the same symptoms, were not doing well on the same recommendations.

That frustration and concern have led researchers like Dr. W .H. Sheldon to rediscover that we are very digestively and hormonally unique. Dr. Sheldon coined the terms ectomorph (similar to S characteristics), endomorph (similar to P characteristics), and mesomorph (similar to B characteristics) for different metabolic types. Think magazine covers illustrating apple, banana, and pear body shapes!

That gives you a little background. Now, let's work on what it all means for you today. The Dietary Needs Assessment (DNA) I use in my practice covers eight physical and emotional genetic differences. Still, the one I'll touch on here—and where you'll get the most energy bang for your labor and time expenditure—is digestion.

P and Px Body Type Oxidizers

Some people are fast oxidizers. That means they have SNPs (and other factors, such as enzyme types/ratios and gut bacteria) that quickly foster their burning through the nutrients in their food. They feel hungry often, and when that hunger hits, it can be fast and furious. In terms of the autonomic nervous system, this is most typically a Parasympathetic Dominant (P or Px Body Type) response.

S and Sx Body Types – Slow Oxidizers

For slow oxidizers, usually those that are Sympathetic Dominant (S or Sx Body Type), their SNPs (and, again, other factors such as enzymes and stress) cause them to respond to food in a way that fosters slower digestion. They can go longer periods without eating, and hunger—when it comes—is more gradual.

Balanced Body Types – Mid-Range Oxidizers

A balanced body type (B) would fall more mid-range between a slow-oxidizer Carbohydrate Body Type and a fast-oxidizer Protein Body Type. Depending upon their second highest number on the Dietary Needs Assessment (P or S), this type would lean more toward one set of traits than the other.

So, now that you know your metabolic type and know a little more about what that means for you physically, how can you use that information to reduce fatigue, increase cognitive functioning, and balance moods?

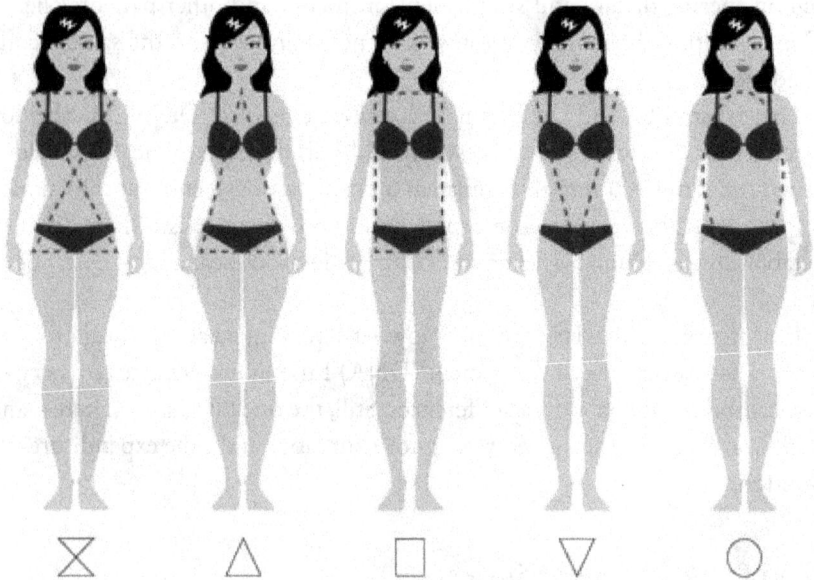

Metabolic Types

Digestion, Campfire Style

First, consider the rate of digestion in terms of feeding a campfire and the macronutrients as fuel. Carbohydrates, especially fruit and raw and cooked non-starchy vegetables, tend to burn (be digested) reasonably rapidly, so they could be considered toothpick fuel or kindling.

Regarding energy production, their relatively quick output of a glucose rise can be helpful, but they don't have much "staying power" energy-wise. In addition, any rapid glucose rises you don't utilize pretty quickly through muscle exertion (sitting at your computer doesn't count!) can get stored as fat and soon leave you feeling hungry again.

This last factor is particularly relevant as P and Px Body Types are highly efficient at energy conservation or, more simply, fat storage. This trait is super important (and indeed crucial to survival!) in times of famine. However, it's not as helpful when food, particularly sugary and refined food, is in ample supply.

S and Sx Body Types—with their combination of fast metabolic rate and genetic propensity to being least efficient at converting food into stored fat—tend toward leanness even when the food supply is abundant.

In camping terms, for a P or Px, burning fruits and vegetables, and even slightly longer burning carbs such as whole grains and starchy vegetables, as primary fuel makes about as much sense as throwing kindling on a fire to keep you warm all night. Theoretically, it works, but it's not a helpful long-term solution.

Protein-rich and fat-rich foods tend to take longer to digest and make their way into your bloodstream. In campfire terms, think of them as a medium-sized branch or log. If you are a P or Px Body Type and have been primarily fueling with fruits, vegetables, and other carbohydrates, you will likely feel hungry often. The grainy, sugary, dried fruit-laden granola and berries you have for breakfast, that loaded baked potato for lunch, and a snack of organic corn chips and salsa will all be rapid work for your strong digestion.

You'll feel some excellent initial blood sugar elevation with the resulting energy, mental clarity, and an increased buoyant mood, but it won't last long. You'll shortly feel hungry again, need to eat to raise your blood sugar levels and, unless you're a more disciplined and sounder-thinking person than I was, it probably won't be steamed, buttered broccoli and grilled tuna you head for, but something more akin to an ultra-processed cookie or fatty, salty snack pack. And soon enough, the pattern starts all over again!

The best and fastest way to break that cycle and gain consistent energy and a fit and comfortable-for-you body size is to start eating real foods to keep your metabolic "fire" more consistently stoked. For Balanced and P or Px Body Types, that generally means reducing—note I didn't say eliminating—carbohydrates (if intake has been too high or too processed) and adding more protein-rich foods and fat to their diet.

It seems counter-intuitive—"I'm a P Body Type, I'm carrying excess body fat, and you want me to eat more fat?"—but it works well in most cases, provided you're eating the correct type of fat.

REST STOP

Time to take a break and digest information!

Take 10 minutes of calm to Rest with the following questions:

- What mistakes have you unknowingly made regarding eating because you were not metabolic-type aware?

- What are you feeling regarding previous styles of eating? Remember to set these questions and answers on a bed of compassion. We make our choices based on what makes the most sense to us at the time.

- What changes do you need to make to avoid repeating those mistakes?

Next, Stop for 10 minutes of quiet (sitting or slowly walking). Keep your mind as clear and open as possible, and just listen. Jot down any responses that may arise.

ROADWORK

Choose the option that most resonates with you. Note the option and your response in your *Trip Log*.

Option 1– Review the sample menu plans tailored to your body type. What is your initial response to the plan? Does it seem manageable? Are you willing to give it a try?

Option 2 – Want to eat even more specifically for your body type? Create a week's menu plan based on your body type and the sample menu ideas in Leg 5. If you want help, you can order a comprehensive set of menu plans and recipes for two weeks' meals for all three body types. You can purchase 101 Recipes for Endless Energy here: https://www.inbalancelm.com/101RecipesforEndlessEnergy.

If you prefer to create your own body-type-specific meals and snacks, go for it!

Natural Eating Plan – P, Px or Protein Body Type

BREAKFAST:

Protein – cleanly-sourced eggs, beef, bison, lamb, poultry (dark meat), wild game, fatty fish (salmon, herring, sardines, anchovies)

Vegetables – raw or cooked, diced veggies in an omelet, poached eggs on steamed spinach, leftover vegetables and meat from the previous night's supper

Fat – butter or coconut oil for cooking

LUNCH:

Large salad – lettuce, cucumber, carrot (in small amounts), celery, parsley, avocado

Optional additions – radish, beet, watercress, kale, green beans, Swiss chard, collards, asparagus, mushrooms, snap peas, artichoke, olives, cauliflower

Dressing – virgin or extra virgin olive oil, avocado oil, coconut oil and apple cider vinegar or lemon juice, herbs, natural seasoning (Spike, Herbamare)

Protein – animal, organic/full fat cheese or, occasionally, vegetable-sourced (nuts, seeds, legumes; minimize peanut and legume intake, especially lima beans, red lentils and soy)

DINNER:

Steamed vegetables – cauliflower, asparagus, green beans

Optional additions – any lunch options (steamed or raw); herbs, lemon juice, butter or olive oil

Protein – cleanly-sourced animal protein such as fish, lamb, turkey, chicken or beef

Carbohydrate – best sources are vegetables, including starchy vegetables like winter squash and sweet potatoes; corn, millet, quinoa, basmati/brown/wild rice and gluten-free oats in limited amounts

Fat – extra virgin olive oil and avocado oil on vegetables, coconut oil for cooking protein, skin on poultry or fat on other meat/fish options, raw avocado

Additional suggestions:

1. Don't drink a lot with meals (dilutes stomach acid and can slow digestion). Have clean water and good herbal teas up to an hour before meals and from 1½ hours after. If you need to have a little liquid with a meal, have small sips of water.
2. Eat approximately equal amounts of vegetables (6 oz.) and protein (6 oz.). Eat until just comfortably full (80/20). Don't overeat. Likewise, do not be left hungry.
3. If possible, do not eat after about 7:00 PM.

Natural Eating Plan - Protein Body Type

Natural Eating Plan – S, Sx or Carbohydrate Body Type

BREAKFAST:

Cooked grain cereal – if best for you, gluten-free   **Fruit –** berries, grapefruit, apple, pear

Well-toasted bread – hearty, sprouted whole grain/seed; again, gluten-free is needed

Fat – butter or nut butter on toast, nuts to top cereal, seeds in bread

LUNCH:

Large salad – lettuce, cucumber, carrot, broccoli, parsley

Optional optimal additions – radish, beet, green onion, watercress, kale, kohlrabi, beet greens, Swiss chard, collards, endive, mustard greens, okra, rutabaga, sprouts

Dressing – virgin or extra virgin olive oil or avocado oil and apple cider vinegar or lemon juice, herbs, natural seasoning (Spike, Herbamare)

Protein – vegetable-sourced (nuts, seeds, legumes, occasional organic, fermented tofu, organic/medium fat cheese; minimize peanut, lentil and soybean intake)

DINNER:

Steamed vegetables – leek, carrot, broccoli, beets

Optional additions – any lunch options (raw or steamed); herbs, lemon juice

Protein – cleanly-sourced animal protein such as lighter fish, turkey or chicken, eggs or Cornish game hen (re: poultry, choose light–breast– over dark–drumstick, back or wings)

Carbohydrate – grains (amaranth, barley, corn, millet, quinoa, brown rice), veggie-loaded baked potato with virgin or extra virgin olive oil and herbs or natural seasoning (Spike, Herbamare). Do not have the baked potato option more than 2-3 times a week.

Fat – extra virgin olive oil or avocado oil on vegetables, avocado

Additional suggestions:

1. Don't drink a lot with meals (dilutes stomach acid and can slow digestion). Have clean water and good herbal teas up to an hour before meals and from 1½ hours after. If you need to have a little liquid with a meal, have small sips of water.
2. Eat a larger amount of vegetables (8 oz.) to protein (4-5 oz.). Eat until just comfortably full (80/20). Don't overeat. Likewise, do not be left hungry.
3. If possible, do not eat after about 7:00 PM.

Natural Eating Plan - Carbohydrate Body Type

Natural Eating Plan – B or Balanced Body Type

Read the Eating Plan for a P (Parasympathetic, Protein Body Type) and an S (Sympathetic, Carbohydrate Body Type). See what most resonates with you as foods you enjoy eating for each meal and find satisfying (hold you from hunger for a time).

Eat those foods in the ratio per the Balance Body Type Plate Portioning graphic shown previously in this Leg. Trial an initial type of foods/ratio for 4-5 days, assessing how you feel physically (energy), mentally (clear thinking), emotionally (balanced moods) and digestion-wise (bloating). For more on the questions, plus a bonus question, check this Leg's Traveller Assistance.

If you rate yourself well in each category, continue eating that way. If not, adjust one factor (add more fat or eat the dark rather than light meat of poultry), give yourself another 4-5 days of eating the adjusted way, and then evaluate again.

Eventually, you will find the suitable types of foods and the ratio of those foods that best suits YOUR body!

TRAVELLER ASSISTANCE – Four Questions to Ask Yourself (over and over again)

One of the most beneficial tools to provide a quick "check-up" of how you are doing on the optimal wellness journey is to regularly ask yourself these four questions:

1. What are my physical energy levels?

2. How is my mental clarity?

3. Are my moods balanced?

4. Do I experience abdominal bloating?

Bonus Question (for longer-term reflection) - Am I easily able to reach and maintain a comfortable-for-me body size?

By regularly reviewing these questions and their answers, you'll easily be able to keep a pulse on how you are doing wellness-wise. And, when answers reveal less-than-optimal responses, you can conduct a Road Block and Traffic Jam evaluation and get back on track sooner rather than later.

A Note About Insulin Resistance

Understanding insulin resistance is critical to understanding metabolic health, how our bodies manage energy, and what to do when this process isn't working efficiently. At least a couple of mainstream and alternative health theories exist on balancing blood sugar levels and ensuring healthy insulin regulation.

First, some background.

Insulin is a hormone that helps our cells absorb glucose (sugar) from the blood, which they use for energy. In a metabolically healthy system, the pancreas releases insulin in response to increased blood sugar levels (such as after eating), and it helps cells take in glucose to be used or stored as energy.

Insulin Resistance occurs when cells in the body respond poorly to insulin. They don't take in glucose as effectively, which means sugar starts to build up in the blood.

Mainstream medicine and many alternative practitioners see the issue as excessive carbohydrate intake and, therefore, advocate an across-the-board no or low-carb approach for anyone dealing with or looking to prevent insulin resistance.

From a bioenergetic perspective, however, insulin resistance can be seen as a cellular energy crisis. When cells do not effectively receive glucose, they are deprived of a fundamental fuel (and are forced to move to backup fuels like fats and proteins). This lack of fuel can impair function and force the body to make more insulin to get glucose into the cells.

Rather than a no-carbohydrate or low-carbohydrate approach, which may initially improve lab results and support the release of excess body fat, the bioenergetic approach would have you address the foundational root causes of that insulin resistance.

That happens, as *Metabolic Health Roadmap* advocates, by looking at the lifestyle factors that would restore metabolic health at a cellular level. Rather than a seemingly quick fix—eliminating or significantly reducing carbohydrate intake—that is long-term going to result in potentially poor cellular energy production and a resulting increase in toxic by-products of burning fatty acids, you restore metabolic health at a cellular level.

And according to bioenergetics, how does one restore that metabolic health?

1. *Optimize your nutrient intake*

- **Ensure adequate macronutrient balance** or, in *Metabolic Health Roadmap* terms, eat the right balance of carbohydrates, protein, and fats for your body type, ensuring stable blood sugar levels and a consistent energy supply.

- **Focus on micronutrients** or, in *Metabolic Health Roadmap* terms, eat foods—and perhaps take supplements—that contain the vitamins and minerals that support cellular functions, especially nutrients like the B vitamins, magnesium, and selenium that help with energy production.

- **Eat high-quality foods** or, in *Metabolic Health Roadmap* terms, follow the Food Foundation and Food Key Guidelines-Leg 3.

2. *Improve stress management*

- **Regular physical activity** or, in *Metabolic Health Roadmap* terms, find joyful exercise that works for your body type-Leg 4.

- **Mindfulness and relaxation techniques** or, in *Metabolic Health Roadmap* terms, Manage Stress for Metabolic Health-Leg 5.

- **Get adequate sleep** or, in *Metabolic Health Roadmap* terms, Rest for Metabolic Health-Leg 4.

3. *Enhance environmental and lifestyle factors*

- **Minimize toxic exposure** or, in *Metabolic Health Roadmap* terms, eat clean food and drink clean water-Leg 3. Also, the quality of personal care and cleaning products should be considered.

- **Regulate light exposure** or, in *Metabolic Health Roadmap* terms, manage light exposure to support proper circadian rhythm functioning-Leg 4.

- **Temperature regulation** or, in *Metabolic Health Roadmap* terms, keeping bedrooms cool at night-Leg 4 and potentially using a sauna to detoxify and relieve stress.

The *Metabolic Health Roadmap* guidelines are more suited to a bioenergetic approach to insulin resistance than an all-inclusive no-carb or low-carb approach.

For an excellent resource in understanding more on the root causes of insulin resistance and, via the bioenergetic approach, resolving those causes and promoting lasting health improvements, check out the Jay Feldman Wellness podcast, in particular, the various studies available in the show notes on any episodes covering insulin resistance.

SOUVENIR

Your Leg Three souvenir, celebrating the time and attention you've been giving to personalized care of yourself, is a fun "body type appropriate" snack. Save it for when you're hungry and choose from some of these options:

Carbohydrate Body Type (S, Sx) — a couple of squares of dark chocolate and a handful of your favorite berries; organic corn chips, salsa, and, if you are dairy-tolerant, a chunk of medium-fat cheese; apple slices with almond butter dip (¼ cup water and ¼ cup almond butter; stir until smooth and well-blended).

Protein Body Type (P, Px) — cleanly-sourced turkey pepperoni slices and carrot sticks; celery filled with almond butter; a chunk of medium-fat cheese and cauliflower pieces; a hard-boiled egg and cucumber slices; cleanly-sourced beef slices, spread with mustard, topped with spinach and rolled; a couple of squares of dark chocolate and a handful of nuts or seeds or a spoonful of nut butter.

Balanced Body Type (B) — Choose a snack from the above-listed Body Types that represents your second-highest score on the Dietary Needs Assessment.

Chapter Twelve

LEG 4 – Move and Rest for Metabolic Health

SUMMARY – Travel Size Version

Where in This Leg, You Will Planfully Incorporate Activity and Foster a Good Night's Sleep!

Diagnostic #3 - Move and Snooze Surveys

For this Leg of your *Metabolic Health Roadmap* journey, we'll once again start by assessing your current state, this time your activity levels and sleep quality.

Activity (that works for you)

We'll look at four "S" words: Simple. Sensible. Safe. Sustainable—fundamental to movement that keeps your body|mind|spirit engaged. Some of these "S" words are favorites of mine that you'll see popping up often, not just because they roll off the tongue with nice-sounding alliteration but because applying them works!

Five Types of Exercise

These five are critical to increased energy and overall health:

- **Functional** – Activity that is a part of your daily living.

- **Endurance** –These "with oxygen" activities are generally longer and more intense and support physical, emotional, and mental wellness in several ways.

- **Strength** – Using body or other weight to build muscle.

- **Balance** – Activities designed to increase balance and prepare you to age well.

- **Flexibility** – Stretching exercises that promote ease of movement.

Which one is most calling your name?

Going Primal

If long-history-of-use activity is more your thing, you'll love and want to incorporate these 6 + 1 Primal moves. They can be done without hitting a gym, investing in expensive equipment, or buying fancy workout gear.

Catch Some ZZZs AND Grab Some Rest (They're Not Necessarily the Same Thing!)

We will examine seven (yup, count them, seven) types of rest: physical, mental, sensory, creative, emotional, social, and spiritual. You will learn what they are, why they're important, and how to put them into practice.

Habits (how you do something is how you do everything)

Here, we'll break down habits into their "seed" components and discover how to grow a good one and how to weed out a bad one.

Chapter Thirteen

LEG 4 – Move and Rest: Getting Started

"Many of the people I work with that are half my age complain that they feel tired all the time. I tell them: 'Look at what you're eating, how much you are exercising, and how much sleep you are getting.'"
David H. Murdock, 98-year-old American businessman and philanthropist

O nce you settle on your optimal fuel intake and regularly feed yourself accordingly, the next step to optimal metabolic health is evaluating how you Make Some Moves (your physical activity) and Catch Some ZZZs (your rest patterns). The proper amounts and types of exercise can be a super helpful tool for all manner of wellness benefits.

Additionally, understanding the importance of good sleep hygiene can help eradicate Road Blocks to increased energy. Knowing the different types of rest that may be needed at various points—and putting them into practice—can provide the clarity and calmness that will make short work of Traffic Jams.

For starters, let's do another check-up, this time, a couple of short surveys: a *Move Survey* and a *Snooze Survey*.

Diagnostic #3 – Move and Snooze Surveys

Movement and rest (including physical sleep) are essential—and often over-looked—keys to increased metabolic health. With Objectivity, Curiosity, and Compassion, complete the two short surveys that follow and review your results.

Move Survey

Answer yes, no, or sometimes to the questions. Give yourself 2 points for a "yes," 1 point for a "sometimes," and 0 points for a "no."

- Do I enjoy being active?

- Are there a range of physical activities that I enjoy doing?

- Do I incorporate functional fitness in my life (taking stairs over the elevator)?

- Do I do activities weekly that elevate my heart rate?

- Do I do activities weekly that make muscles stronger?

- Do I do activities weekly that increase my flexibility?

- Do I do activities that get me outdoors?

- Do I participate in activity with others?

- Do I have a type of activity I do on my own?

If you scored 13–18:
You're a "move it" maestro! Stick with your activity plan!
If you scored 7-12:
You may be intermittently active. What resonates with you in this Leg? You can begin to incorporate that as an Action Goal.
If you scored 1-6:
You're likely relatively inactive. If so, carefully read the information in this Leg and begin to incorporate small but regular amounts of the different types of activity (one type at a time!)!

Snooze Survey

Answer yes, no, or sometimes to the questions. Give yourself 2 points for a "yes," 1 point for a "sometimes," and 0 points for a "no."

- Do I avoid eating ultra-processed grains and sugars before bed?

- Do I eat a high-protein snack a couple of hours before bed?

- Do I avoid caffeine after about 2 pm?

- Do I sleep in complete darkness?

- Do I keep my bedroom cool at night?

- Do I avoid TV/other screens for at least an hour before bed?

- Do I read something calming or contemplative before bed?

- Do I journal before bed?

- Do I get to bed before 11:00 pm?

- Do I keep my bed only for sleeping or romance?

- If needed, do I use melatonin, L-tryptophan or 5-HTP?

If you scored 15–22:
You're likely a stellar sleeper! Keep up the excellent work.

If you scored 8-14:
You may be an on-again/off-again good sleeper. Please look at what resonates in this Leg and apply the appropriate steps.

If you scored 1-7:
You're likely a relatively poor sleeper. If so, take particular note of this Leg's information and schedule as many as possible of the steps (one at a time!) into your sleep hygiene practice until sleep habits and benefits improve.

Have you got your scores? Pay particular attention to high scores (areas you can use for Habit Hitching—more on that later) and low scores (indicating areas that could use some help). With both scenarios, pay attention to what resonates as you read through this Leg.

OK . . . let's move on (pun intended!).

Chapter Fourteen

LEG 4 - Activity that Works for YOU

"Pick a type of movement that not only strengthens your muscles, lungs, and heart ... but that brings joy to your soul!"

Brenda Wollenberg

Information Centre

We often think of movement, activity, or exercise as something that burns calories. It is a method of compensating for food intake. A "calories in/calories out" type of math. A mentality of, "I ate this; therefore, I must do this many laps or spin classes or weight sessions or ... "

First, simply moving your body has less initial impact than many other factors on things like body shape and size. We know so much more now about how different body types burn different types of fuel. We better understand concepts like what foods and factors contribute to slowing metabolism or fostering insulin resistance. There is much research being done in the field of genetics (the body shape and size you are "wired for") and, beyond that, epigenetics (a quick reminder: looking at the influences on genes—both behavior and environment—that affect the ways your genes work) that is giving an increased understanding of the impact of factors such as food, activity, thought and hormones on our body shape and size.

Therefore, realize that should one of your Faith Goals be to shed excess body fat, I'm not asking you to consider movement and activity as a primary method of that fat release. In many people, exercise plays a relatively minor role in body size, smaller, for example, than the fuel mix they eat, the amount and quality of sleep they get, how they handle stress, AND how they feel about and speak about their body. Instead, I'm asking you to incorporate regular bouts of various types of movement for multiple other reasons. Movement has massive amounts of impact on mood and cognitive functioning. It can be utilized as a stress management tool. As a factor in gaining metabolic health, it can play a significant role in vitality and invigoration.

The Exercise/Metabolic Health Connection

So, if exercise and movement are not primarily about weight loss, how *do* we view physical activity in a health-supporting way? First, look at exercise's dynamic interaction with metabolic health. The relationship between exercise and metabolic health is bidirectional; improvement in one can lead to benefits in the other.

Let's start with how improved metabolic health can enhance your exercise abilities and outcomes:

1. **Increased energy efficiency** - When your metabolic health improves, your body can better utilize energy sources during activity. When cells are well-regulated in insulin sensitivity and muscles do a great job of glucose uptake, you'll experience sustained energy levels, critical factors in endurance and performance.

2. **Better muscle function** - Metabolic health involves effectively delivering nutrients and oxygen to muscles. Improved muscle health and performance can, in turn, improve strength, capacity, and endurance.

3. **Reduced fatigue** - Metabolic health helps you better manage lactic acid levels and can delay fatigue onset, improving exercise tolerance and performance.

Next, increased exercise enhances metabolic health:

1. **Improved insulin sensitivity** - We're back to insulin sensitivity. Regular exercise, in a type that suits your genetics, can support insulin signaling and increase muscle cells' sensitivity to insulin, a crucial factor in preventing metabolic conditions like type 2 diabetes.

2. **Enhanced cardiovascular and lymphatic function** - Among other benefits, exercise can strengthen the heart, improve circulation, and

enhance the movement of lymph fluid through the lymphatic system, which is a passive system not pumped by the heart. This movement is vital in transporting nutrients to cells and removing cellular waste material, which can support improved metabolic health.

3. **Reduction in visceral fat** - While every body is different and will have a healthy percentage of body fat at its most comfortable size, regular physical activity can help reduce excess body fat, particularly the more problematic-for-health visceral fat. Excess amounts of visceral or intra-abdominal fat, found in the spaces around many of our internal organs, can be a key contributing factor to metabolic syndrome and related metabolic disorders.

Understanding the reciprocal relationship between metabolic health and exercise underscores the importance of incorporating physical activity into daily life. Now, how the heck do you go about doing that?

The Four "S"s of Movement

I'm suggesting exercise be viewed through my four "S" lenses:
1. Simple

2. Sensible

3. Safe

4. Sustainable

#1 Simple

Most of us already have an overflowing plate of activities, commitments, and relationships and aren't looking to fill that up further. (For more on Sustainability, Check out the 4th "S" below and this section's Travel Assistance.)

As you review the movement suggestions to follow, pay particular attention to those that seem easy to you, both in terms of the type of activity and incorporating them into your current life scenario.

#2 Sensible

Following hot on the sneaker-clad heels of "simple" comes "sensible." You've probably already got the message that I'm big on dreams, vision, and faith. I have a significant life mission and plans to reach many people with a metabolic health revolution message. I also have a large family to whom I'm committed to having lots of time-rich and deep relationships.

That means my movement needs to be woven through my other significant life goals in a way that doesn't derail those plans. To be sensible and integrated, it needs to support and increase the likelihood that those dreams come to fruition.

So, I power walk with my husband, canoe with good friends, and stroller walk/explore the neighborhood with my young grandchildren. I did Tabata (a form of HIIT—high-intensity interval training) for several years, often alongside my youngest daughter who was also an eager Tabata participant.

The bottom line is that rather than being a jarring and impractical interruption to your life, where can exercise complement you and your dreams?

#3 Safe

Don't get me wrong. I'm all for pushing myself physically at times. Witness running multiple half-marathons, hikes down icy trails into the Grand Canyon, portage-filled canoe trips, 21-day hot yoga class challenges, and initially out-side-my-comfort-zone scuba diving. But I always assess what my body is saying and can handle at any given point.

I make sure I have a team of healthcare professionals (a medical doctor, natur-opathic physician, massage therapist, chiropractor, osteopath, acupuncturist, physiotherapist) available to help in that assessment and, if needed, for recovery. And I almost always listen when my body says to slow down or take a break! As Jonathan Bailor—the lead researcher on the most extensive scientific analysis of health and fitness ever conducted and inspiration for these 4 "S"s—says, copious amounts of heavy or extreme exercise are not all that helpful.

So, not only are unsafe-for-you types of activity unwise in the long term for taking proper care of your body, mind, and spirit, but they aren't all that useful, even in the short term.

#4 Sustainable

By sustainable, I'm looking at several factors. First, is it simple, sensible, and safe enough to be a longer-term activity you'll enjoy and follow through with? And secondly, is it trackable? While I want your movement to be enjoyable, it's also helpful—as most of us can talk ourselves out of anything—if you can track how often you move and the duration and intensity (keep reading for more on amounts to aim for).

The Four "S"s of Movement

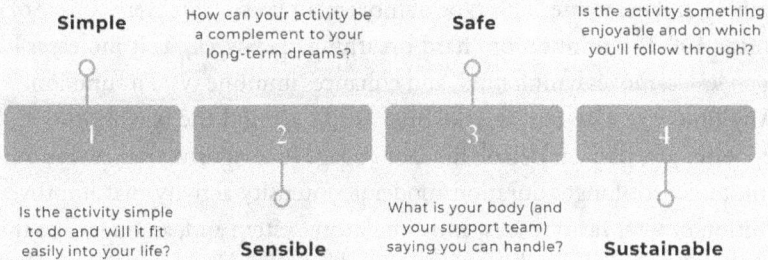

	Simple	How can your activity be a complement to your long-term dreams?		Safe	Is the activity something enjoyable and on which you'll follow through?
1		2	3		4
Is the activity simple to do and will it fit easily into your life?		Sensible	What is your body (and your support team) saying you can handle?		Sustainable

The Four "S"s of Movement

Five Types of Exercise (Move Your Body, Make Some Muscle!)

#1. Functional

Start with functional fitness. As the name implies, this is a handy, purposeful, and valuable exercise that is a regular part of daily living!

- Walking rather than driving to the corner store

- Taking the stairs instead of the elevator

- Weeding the garden

- Vigorous vacuuming

- Chasing a toddler around for an afternoon

- Running up and down the stairs on laundry day

Every chance you get, put thought and energy into the practical activity that is a part of your day. Move with intent, joy, and vitality, and—for little time and money expenditure—you'll reap many rewards!

#2 Endurance

Endurance fitness activities are aerobic—with oxygen—and increase both breathing and heart rate. This type of movement is excellent every couple of days (aim for 100-150 minutes of "hard breathing" per week) as it increases blood oxygen levels, moves lymph fluid, and enhances immune system function.

Any time you play tennis, take brisk walks around the neighborhood, bike ride, swim, jog, play pickleball, hike, or engage in a vigorous dance session, you are on target for longer-duration/moderate-intensity activity that improves the condition of your heart, lungs, and circulatory system and, among other things, can help prevent diabetes, heart disease, and colon and breast cancers.

Also, because many types of endurance exercise can be done outside, you have the potential to benefit from breathing fresh air and, through sunlight on skin exposure, enhancing your vitamin D production.

#3 Strength

Muscular strength plays a significant role in quality of life:
- Strong muscles make everyday activities easier

- Strong muscles support posture and balance and can prevent falls

- Strong muscles support independence

Strength training for major muscle groups (legs, upper body) should occur at least two days/week on alternating days. Be sure to start with minimal amounts of weight, and don't hold your breath. Breathe out as you lift or push, and breathe in as you relax. In addition, if you're new to strength training, get input from trained personnel (sports trainer, physical therapist) on how to lift safely.

Some options for ways to add strength activities to your week:
- Lift weights, your body weight, or carry groceries

- Wall push-ups, gripping a tennis ball, arm curls

- Resistance band exercises

#4 Balance

Activity that enhances balance is essential for several reasons, the primary of which is to prevent falls. Falls can have serious consequences at any age, particularly among older people.

Note that balance exercises do not have to be complicated, and many lower-body strength activities also improve balance. Consider these options:

- Stand on one foot or stand from a seated position

- Walk a beam or log or do a "heel-toe" walk

- Practice yoga or Tai Chi, a "moving meditation" where you slowly shift body movement

As with other types of activity, start slowly with balance exercises. Use support (e.g. a wall, a fence, a friend) when beginning. Check with your healthcare practitioner if you are still determining if a particular balance activity is for you.

#5 Flexibility

The primary way to increase flexibility is with properly done stretching. Stretching of this type has many benefits:

- Increased freedom of movement

- Increased ease in performing daily activities

- An additional method to measure overall fitness

There are many ways to enhance flexibility and different body parts on which to concentrate stretches. Work with a personal trainer or do online searches—from well-regarded sites—to find level-appropriate (beginner, expert) types of these stretches:

- An inner thigh stretch

- A back stretch exercise

- An ankle stretch

- A back-of-leg stretch

Breathe normally throughout your stretching activity. Stretch once muscles are warm (after endurance and strength exercises). Avoid stretching to the point of pain. And, for flexibility purposes—as opposed to preventing stiffness—be sure to hold the stretch for a minimum of 30 seconds.

6 + 1 Essential Movements (Taking it Primal)

If even thinking about hitting the gym, playing a sport, lifting weights, or taking up dance makes you begin to break out in nervousness (or hives!), fear not.

What if Everyday Movement Counted as Exercise?

There is a way to get massive wellness benefits simply by ensuring your regular functional fitness includes these 6 + 1 essential movements. Who knew that fitness could be simple, sensible, safe, and sustainable?

1. Squat – Use Proper Squat Form

Plant both feet firmly on the ground. Bend your legs to lower your body. Keep chest up, lower back straight. Make sure your knees never go in front of your toes. Squat several times a week (while gardening or playing with children).

2. Lunge – Use Proper Lunge Form

Move one leg to step forward and bend while the other leg remains stationary, such as when stepping over a log. When hiking, where lunges are required, or when playing catch with a ball or frisbee, put this into practice.

3. Push – Use Proper Push-up Form

Pushing weight away from you or pushing your center of mass away from the ground (push-up) is a movement that can be used to push yourself off the floor or a box onto a shelf. If you are new to push-ups, start with wall push-ups, then move to push-ups with your hands on a counter or couch, then move to the floor on your hands and knees and, finally, on your hands and feet.

4. Pull – Use Proper Pull-up Form

The opposite of pushing is pulling a weight toward your body. You can start up an older-style pull-cord motorboat or lawn mower. When picking apples or blackberries, pull a branch to grab the fruit.

5. Twist – Use a Rotational Movement

Not just moving forward or to the side but using a twisting movement. The best ways to incorporate this primal move are to reach across your body, throw a ball, or incorporate loose twisting movement while walking or running.

6. Bend – Use Proper Deadlift Form

Bend the torso over by hinging hips. Think of the movement needed to pick up a baby off the ground or lift a heavy suitcase. This movement can be problematic for many people with lower back pain; check with your healthcare practitioner before doing so. Keeping a slight bend in the knee when performing bends can help, and lift with your legs, not your back.

+1. Gait, The Ultimate of All Movement

A loose-limbed, easy-moving gait can incorporate all 6 Primal movements. Practice it often!

+1 - GAIT: THE ULTIMATE OF ALL MOVEMENT

WALKING, JOGGING, SPRINTING

Running to catch the bus, taking a walk in the park with your dog, playing tag with the kids.

GAIT

PULLING, LUNGING, TWISTING

Gait is the most often used movement in our daily life, on its own or with other moves like jumping or crawling.

Gait: The Ultimate Movement

REST STOP

Time to take a break and digest information!

Take 10 minutes of calm to Rest with the following questions:

1. What types of activity, if any, do I currently do regularly?

2. What type of activity do I currently need the most?

Next, Stop for 10 minutes of quiet (sitting or slowly walking). Keep your mind as clear and open as possible, and just listen. Jot down any responses that may arise.

ROADWORK

Choose the option that most resonates with you. Note the option and your response in your *Trip Log*.

Option 1 – With what you believe to be your most needed type of activity in mind, begin to get curious about why that activity has not been regularly occurring:

- Do you have a history of that type of activity? If so, what were your experiences?

- If you have been avoiding certain types of activity, can you dig beneath the behavior and ask yourself why not engaging in that activity has made sense to you?

Option 2 – If you are ready and able to begin incorporating one new type of activity into your week, ask yourself:

- Where can I add small amounts of that activity to my current schedule?

- How can I make that addition as simple as possible?

- What am I going to do to track that activity?

And, then, for additional support in incorporating your new activity, read on to this Leg's Traveller Assistance on Seed Habits.

TRAVELLER ASSISTANCE – Seed Habits

In the next Traveller Assistance, we'll examine the best way to grow a good habit, but before we do that, let's discuss the concept of Seed Habits.

Often, when we read a new and motivating book, attend a weekend workshop, or listen to an exciting lifestyle podcast, we decide to make changes—revolutionary changes, life-altering changes. And we decide the best way to make such a monumental change is with monumental action.

Unfortunately, that's not how most of us grow. Big change actions usually fizzle out into big change failures. The rare individual starts one day as a mustard seed (Look it up. It's tiny.) and grows to a full-sized mustard plant the following week (Look it up. It's big!).

Most of us need to grow incrementally, with:

- Seed Habits

- Sprout Habits

- Sapling Habits . . .

. . . before we hit Sequoia Habits.

The giant sequoia is the largest tree in the world in terms of volume. It has an immense trunk and a vast spread. However, like most great, glorious, massive objects, ideas, and behaviors, it starts as a seed. So, how do you translate that slow but steady and incremental growth concept into metabolic health language? You find that tackling the path of least resistance and incorporating small Seed Habits into each wellness area resonates with you.

What Do Seed Habits Look Like?

Seed Habits have four primary characteristics (in fact, most of them will probably remind you of the "S" words I gave you for movement criteria!). Here they are in our Seed Habit Checklist:

- **Small (in the amount of time they take):** Initially, begin your new, soon-to-be habit action with a mustard seed's worth of time. Set aside 2-5 minutes. Put the timer on. Do it.

- **Simple (as in one action):** Don't revamp your total bedtime routine. Instead, add one new object (lavender pillow spray) or remove one old behavior (being on your phone until the lights are out).

- **Sensible (as in convenient and not-too-unfamiliar):** Pick an action without a steep learning curve that doesn't jar your sensibilities. Don't, for example, try learning three new sleep meditations in 5 minutes.

- **Sustainable (it's trackable, and there's an 80% chance you'll keep it up):** Is it easy to tell if you've done/not done the action? Can you measure the number of steps, eyeball the amount of protein you ate, and note how many chapters you read? And are you feeling pretty good about the habit? That's sustainable.

When you think about making a change, please review the Seed Habit checklist. Your body, mind, and spirit will thank you!

Chapter Fifteen

LEG 4 - Sleep - Catch Some ZZZs

"Rest is the most underused, chemical-free, safe, and effective alternative therapy available to us."

Dr. Saundra Dalton-Smith

INFORMATION CENTRE

For much of my life, and for various body, mind, and spirit reasons, rest has often been a two-step forward, one-step backward dance for me. Luckily, it has been more like three or four steps forward before a backward step in recent years! That progress makes me very happy and has enhanced my energy levels, too!

Once again, in looking at Rest, we're going simple and helping you understand an easy **What** (a description of each of the seven types of rest we will be looking at), **Why** (that type of rest is essential, its benefits), and **How** (to *best fit* that type of rest into your life).

And we'll start this section's Information Centre by, right out of the gate, busting the myth that sleep and rest are the same thing. They're not! There are, in fact, at least seven types of rest.

Physical rest, or sleep, is generally top-of-mind rest and is often the only rest we consider.

Instead, I'll encourage you to consider six other types of rest for improved metabolic health and endless energy. With that complement, you'll cover a fuller body|mind|spirit range and be able to tap into many energy-producing parts of who you are.

For those of you who are research-focused, I've used information from an internal medicine doctor, Dr. Saundra Dalton-Smith, as the foundation for much of this Leg's thoughts. For a quick review of her findings, check out her TED Talk.

However, before digging into rest, let's examine the relationship between this topic and metabolic health. I'll drill down into the information in pertinent "rest" categories, but let's begin with a bird's eye view.

As with many of this book's leg topics, the relationship between sleep or rest and metabolic health is bidirectional. Improvement in one often leads to benefits in the other.

A couple of the ways that improved metabolic health can lead to better sleep or rest outcomes are:

Enhanced hormonal balance - Metabolic health influences the balance of many hormones. Regarding sleep and rest, improved melatonin production and well-regulated cortisol production can lead to sounder sleep.

Decreased inflammation - Improved metabolic health is often associated with reduced systemic inflammation. Because inflammation can interfere with sleep, either causing discomfort or altering neurotransmitter systems involved in sleep regulation, better metabolic health has the potential to enhance sleep and rest.

Reciprocally, better sleep can support better metabolic health:

Hormone regulation - In particular, sufficient quality sleep plays a role in properly regulating appetite hormones like leptin and ghrelin. When leptin and ghrelin regulation is optimal, hunger messages are appropriately timed, satiety is appropriately reached, and the risks of overeating and diseases that arise from overeating are minimized.

Reduction of stress and inflammatory markers - Restorative sleep reduces levels of stress and inflammation in the body, both factors in poor metabolic outcomes. The body better regulates stress hormones and can reduce the levels of inflammatory cytokines, a signaling molecule that promotes inflammation.

Now, let's translate those science-backed foundations into some real-life practical steps.

Brenda's Classic Client

I enjoy working with a wide range of interesting, funny, intelligent, hard-working, giving, thoughtful, and kind clients who walk through my office door or appear on my Zoom screen. They are all unique and complex individuals I love partnering with in body|mind|spirit detective work to discover and resolve factors contributing to presenting concerns.

However, there are usually common threads of wellness complaints related to that uniqueness. While excess body fat and some emotional distress (low mood, irritability, anxiety) are highly customary, probably the most widespread health concern is fatigue.

Most of my clients' intake forms express concern about lack of energy, tiredness, insufficient stamina to accomplish necessary tasks, exhaustion, weariness, or lethargy.

Indeed, lack of or poor-quality sleep plays a role. Many of my clients also list insomnia as an issue. Beyond that, though, I've discovered over the years that a lack of sleep and rest has led to the fact that my high-achieving, high-producing, "I've got this," handle-everything clients are also chronically fatigued and burned out!

Brenda's Classic Way of Supporting Her Clients to Wellness

Once we've tackled food (remember, energy trumps everything, and eating real food, per your body type, is the place to start!) and begin the gentle implementation of appropriate and regular movement, the next stop is looking at physical rest and sleep hygiene, the type of rest we'll spend the most amount of time exploring.

#1 Physical Rest

This is the aspect that usually first comes to mind when we think about rest.

What it is: Quality physical rest—sleep—is crucial to reaching and maintaining optimal health. Duration and depth of the various sleep cycles all play a role in the value of our sleep time.

Why it matters: First, poor sleep leads to more stress. Our increased workloads and insufficient understanding of the importance of sleep and the factors that impact sleep mean that we are getting less sleep and suffering more stress. Increased stress means increased cortisol production by the adrenal glands. That, in turn, leads to various health challenges, including decreased melatonin production and, therefore, reduced protection from cancer and increased accumulation of fat, particularly abdominal fat.

PHYSICAL REST

Put it into Practice:

- Set and keep a regular bedtime
- Establish a bedtime routine
- Turn off the lights
- Minimize EMFs
- Don't take yourself too seriously

Get quality sleep!

Physical Rest - Put it into Practice

Secondly, key appetite hormones are affected by sleep. Leptin, which works to decrease appetite, and ghrelin, which increases feelings of hunger, are both impacted by insufficient sleep. Leptin is reduced—upping your appetite—and ghrelin is increased—along with your feelings of hunger. Where food is readily available, increased appetite can contribute to obesity, especially:

- For Protein Body Types who are very efficient at fat storage.

- For all body types when, as is often the case, the increased appetite isn't necessarily directed toward protein-rich foods and vegetables!

How to best put it into practice:
Set and keep an appropriate bedtime. The refreshment and restoration that come to the body and mind during a good night's sleep are essential to wellness.

Set a reasonable bedtime—most adults need 7-8 hours of sleep to be well rested, and even more in winter months. Note, too, that Protein Body Types generally need more sleep than Carbohydrate Body Types.

Regardless of body type, keep sleep regular, as changing sleep/wake-up times can disrupt body rhythms. If there are shifts, for example, due to holidays, weekends, or work schedules, try to keep sleep/wake-up times the same by 30-60 minutes.

Establish a bedtime routine. Preparing mind, body, and soul for bedtime is critical to restful sleep. Your personality and circumstances will determine routines, but suggestions include:

1. A warm bath

2. Personal reading

3. Quiet family game time

4. Fresh air

5. Meditation (maybe asking some of the age-old contemplative questions such as: for what moment today am I most grateful, and for what moment am I least grateful?)

6. A small snack 1-2 hours before bed (a bit of protein and fruit can help with melatonin and serotonin production)

7. Diffusing lavender essential oil

8. Cool bedroom

To add to sleep time peace, rather than carrying problems over to the next day, make it a habit to find a resolution to the conflict or, at the least, before bedtime, schedule a time soon to attend to that conflict.

Turn off the lights! In days gone by, sunset and the resultant growing darkness allowed melatonin production, a hormone that helps with many functions, including sleep. With growing levels of light pollution comes the need to ensure your room is as dark as possible at night. Place room-darkening shades on windows and move any light-producing electronics or night light out of your bedroom. If need be, wear a sleep mask.

Minimize EMFs. All of us can be negatively impacted by the electrical pollution produced by electrical appliances and electronic wireless devices. Clear your bedroom of computers, cell phones, and handheld landlines, avoid electric blankets and water beds (are those even a thing anymore?), and revert to a battery-operated alarm clock. EMFs negatively impact melatonin production, which, in turn, leads to a myriad of health challenges—sleep disturbance is one of them.

Don't take yourself too seriously . . . she says as she has just finished talking about things like sourcing clean food, reducing your sugar intake, and trying to find time to be active regularly! Why the admonition to laugh a bit? While laughter does indeed burn calories (a consideration for slow-oxidizer Parasympathetic Body Types), the main reason laughter plays a role in helping keep wellness and body size at a healthy level is because laughter helps counteract the effects of stress in the body.

Cortisol, a "fight or flight" hormone produced by the adrenal glands, is necessary and helpful for specific situations. Its levels should be high in the morning to boost your energy to start your day or if you are being chased by a tiger (an unlikely but highly stressful situation). In the latter case, you'd appreciate the increased flow of glucose, protein, and fat and the fact that cortisol will move out of your tissues for immediate use in your extremities. Note, as well, that when it comes to your brain, emotional and physical pain or stress are almost the same. So, while I am talking about "tigers," similar bodily responses can also occur when you are worried about paying that month's bills or are experiencing a serious relationship challenge.

As the day progresses, your cortisol levels should take natural drops and then level slightly at different times until they reach their lowest point at bedtime. During a proper, restful, deep sleep, cortisol levels rise to a natural high at the beginning of the next day.

Because of today's increased environmental and emotional stress levels, however, most of us have too much or erratic levels of cortisol and, therefore, are susceptible to conditions that high levels of the hormone are linked with, storage of visceral fat (surrounding abdominal organs), diabetes, insomnia, heart disease, lowered immune system functioning and depression. Laughter can be a valuable tool to keep cortisol at healthy levels.

#2 Mental Rest

AKA giving your brain a break.

What it is: Before moving on to mental rest, the second of the seven types of rest we'll cover, I'll take a minute or two to sidestep and foster awareness that these are not isolated types of rest. It's not like you need to figure out one that is deficit and work only on that one at the expense of the others. Just like we don't exert only one type of body|mind|spirit energy in any given situation and concentrate on strengthening that.

We're not a body, or a mind, or a spirit. We're interconnected. Note to self: review the Traveller Assistance on the Broccoli Rubber Band Exercise in Leg 1.

A Mt. Everest Tale

Take, for example, a very physical activity—climbing to a base camp at Mt. Everest—like our middle son, Joel, did with his friend, Doug, several years ago. That took massive amounts of physical energy. However, mental energy played a significant role, as did social energy. Joel and Doug needed to interact well, support, and calm each other throughout the trip, especially when they got lost in a whiteout blizzard.

And when Joel's mom—me!—later heard about their near-death experience, it used up a lot of her emotional and spiritual energy. So, just like energy expenditure is interconnected, consider these types of rest not in isolation but in an interconnected way.

Why it matters: Rest for the mind is a quieting of the rational, thinking, planning, and "figuring out" part of our brain. A mind always on the go has an extreme need for this type of rest. Mental rest helps calm what is often called "monkey brain," a way of constantly looking for ways to solve the problems of your household, workplace, or the world! A continually racing brain doesn't allow one to experience the benefits of mental rest. There is no time for mindfulness. There isn't a lot of ability to be thinking about being grateful. That means this type of rest is essential for allowing the rational brain to down-regulate to better pay attention to what is happening in the body and spirit.

How to best put it into practice:

1. *Use practical self-scheduling tools.* Set a timer on your clock to break up the parts of your day that require large amounts of mental energy. I often do 48/12s with a timer, giving me 48 minutes of concentrated work (no phone, social media notification, or email alerts) and then 12 minutes of downtime to make a cup of tea, do some stretching, walk barefoot in my backyard, take a bathroom break, stare out the window and give my computer-focused eyes a rest.

2. *Support the parasympathetic part of your autonomic nervous system.* Anyone who suffers from mental overdrive and the need for additional mental rest will find it essential—and sometimes challenging—to support the parasympathetic (rest and recuperate and restore) part of the autonomic nervous system to help balance out the sympathetic (flight, fight, freeze or fawn) part. Note that we'll cover some simple and effective ways of doing so in the next Leg, Manage Stress for Metabolic Health.

#3 Sensory Rest

Next, let's take a took at the overload of what you see, hear, and smell.

What it is: Think back to the last time you were in the country, perhaps camping or backpacking. And I mean out in the country, where there are no street lights, flashing neon signs, or glowing marquees!

Basically, out where it is dark. That's what I mean by sensory rest. Before electricity and readily available light sources, this is how we lived.

Why it matters: Today, with ambient light, constant screen activity, noise pollution in every household, street, and city, and a regular olfactory assault of cooking, cleaning, and manufacturing odors, whether or not we are aware of it, our senses are bombarded with sights, sounds and smells all day, every day.

We have grown accustomed to certain light, noise, and odor levels. That doesn't, however, mean that it is good for us. If left unchecked, ongoing sensory overload can lead to—you guessed it—sensory overload syndrome.

Sensory rest goes a long way to combat ambient light, the blue light of device screens, and the onslaught of noise and odors that can overwhelm the senses.

How to best put it into practice:

Take regular breaks to close your eyes or use noise-cancelling devices (earplugs or headphones). Schedule a device-free time (especially right before bed). Consider "vacations" from electronics, be they partial or whole days (or scary as it may seem, more extended periods such as a week).

#4 Creative Rest

Here, I'm going to deviate a bit from what Dr. Dalton-Smith talks about in that I see both the need she mentions for a rest *from* creativity, as well as a rest *in* creativity, depending upon your situation. So, this is where you get to, sorry, be creative.

What it is: Taking a break from being creative OR making room for creativity.

Why it matters: Creative rest is whatever awakens the child-like wonder in you and brings some joy. Sometimes, our work environment requires a lot of creative output. If that's you, creative rest can look like increasing joy by being less innovative, giving that part of your brain a break.

And for some of us, creative rest is getting a little more creative.

White Chocolate, American Buttercream Frosted Naked Wedding Cakes

"How," you might ask, "Does a heading like that fit into a section on rest?" Good question!

Our oldest daughter and her fiancé asked if I'd make their wedding cake a few years ago. I was like, ah no. I bake organic muffins and whole-grain cookies. Not white chocolate wedding cakes that take more sugar in one go around than I generally use in 3 years! But I started to get intrigued. I spent hours on Pinterest and YouTube and looking at recipes with Rachel. I got excited. I thought, "Maybe I can do this!"

Even though the task was slightly nerve-racking—they were having a "high-end" wedding at a beautiful vintage location, and I did not want to screw this up—I loved trying different recipes, chatting with a fantastic baker friend of mine to learn about the "chemistry" of baking, and our kids loved the six months of practice cakes that they got to sample.

And guess what I discovered? I tackled a new thing. I used a different part of my brain. I got stimulated and excited and succeeded at making something really beautiful! My confidence grew so much that I baked a wedding cake for Joel and his wife, Joanna, a couple of summers ago and, more recently, one for our youngest daughter, Rebekah, and her husband, Ryan. New flavors. New ingredients. New creative rest!

How to best put it into practice: First, determine if you need a rest *from* creativity or a rest *in* creativity. Is there too much inventiveness in your life? Give yourself a breather. Ensure your weekends and downtime include something other than making something fresh and original. There should be no birthing of new projects and nothing requiring creative juices to flow.

For those who realize a need for more creativity, try this. Take a minute and close your eyes. Deep breath in, deep breath out. Put on your 6-year-old, 10-year-old, or 14-year-old hat. During that season of your life, what creatively brought you joy? Music? Pottery? Baking? Whatever it is, start making room to do that again!

#5 Emotional Rest

Most of my female clients find that examining emotional rest hits strikingly close to home.

What it is: Whether we agree with it or not, emotional giving (serving, placating, people-pleasing) is often at the core of a woman's upbringing and expression of self. Emotional rest entails taking a break from that giving.

Why it matters: "Sure, I can do that," or "Yes, I can be there to help," or "I've got it," roll off our lips almost without thinking. We don't take the time to consider a request (to realize that saying "Yes" to one thing always means saying "No" to another—and that "another" thing is often your family or your self-care), to determine if the needed response is in our physical, mental or emotional capacity or whether—even if it is within our means—we want to do that thing!

If "emotional rest" is loudly calling your name, it may be time for a vacation from saying "Yes." Emotional rest is often a high priority for those in helping/supporting/serving professions, but it can be a necessary self-care exercise for anyone.

How to best put it into practice: One of the best and simplest ways to put emotional rest into practice is to buy time before responding to requests. For "Yes, absolutely," substitute the phrase "Thanks for considering me for this. I'll think about it and respond later today!" Or "That is a wonderful opportunity; let me check with my partner/family to see what we have planned, and then I'll get back to you."

As I've mentioned, you are the best authority on yourself. Give yourself time to listen to what you—all of you—are saying. Pay attention to what happens physically, emotionally, and spiritually in your body, mind, and spirit when a request comes in. Ask yourself if what is being suggested for you is something you'd love or would bring you joy (noting that serving can absolutely bring joy!), and then act accordingly.

Recognize that this will sometimes entail saying "No." Stand in front of a mirror and practice saying that word if necessary. No explanations. No "ifs," "ands," or "buts." Just "No."

#6. Social Rest

Whether we lean more toward being an introvert or an extrovert, at some point, we all need a rest from social activity.

What it is: Note that, as mentioned, these types of energy use/rest required don't operate in isolation. Often, the need for social rest and the emotional rest just covered are connected.

What does social rest look like? Rest from social engagement, sometimes totally and on a retreat or weekend alone, sometimes from certain people. In some of my programs, participants do a fair amount of work on relationships. We examine issues such as the health of a relationship and how to produce increased depth. We also look at "extra grace required" friends and relationships, which are challenging but produce significant growth in us.

I'm not saying that everyone in your life should be easy to get along with, meet all your needs, and fulfill all your longings. Different types of relationships require different types and amounts of energy from us. One of the best things we can do is to recognize and even note, on pen and paper, where our different relationships lie on a continuum.

Some are likely "give-and-take" friendships. On life's journey, you are at about the same spot on the road, spiritually, emotionally, and mentally. You have heated discussions, and you help each other out. While one may be in a funk or on an upswing at a different time than you, overall, you are well-paced.

You'll also have friends who are mentors and guides. They are ahead of you on the road, as it were, perhaps just in a particular life category or two (parenting, for example, or business building). Still, you mostly learn from them and grow from *their* input.

And I'm imagining you'll have a few friends who are either further behind you in life's journey—where you're doing a lot of supporting, teaching, and giving—or they're simply those "extra grace required" friends, somewhat like a thorn in your side, but whose behaviors give you a lot of room for reflection, growth, and the ability to practice healthy responses or boundary setting.

Why it's important: Proper social rest allows one to better hang out with the people who restore and revive you when needed; minimize or avoid hanging out with the people who tax or deplete or exhaust you; and maybe even allow for simply hanging out with yourself. Social rest brings grounding as we can become too expansive or spread out with all the people's needs, energies, and personalities in our lives. Sometimes, one needs to draw inward, pull back to yourself, regroup, and then be able to start up again and be more solid in who you are.

How to best put it into practice:

1. *Determine your personality* type, such as whether you're naturally introverted or extroverted. This will give you a big clue about what type of social rest you need.

2. *List people in the three categories I mentioned*, or draw a picture of your life road. Place yourself on the road and then write in the names of people who are a) at the same place, b) ahead of you, that you're reaching out for input/learning, and c) those behind you, that you're reaching out to help along. See how you feel about each of those categories. Determine if specific people should be inside or outside your time/energy circle for a season at least.

#7. Spiritual Rest

Spiritual rest is a place to move beyond the physical and emotional.

What it is: As Dr. Dalton-Smith says in her talk, spiritual rest is "A place that is greater than yourself and your day-to-day routine." A place that allows us to have a deep sense of belonging. A place where we feel unconditionally accepted and loved. For those with some faith practice, it will be intertwined with their understanding of a higher power, the infinite or the divine. Those of secular belief may resonate more with a sense of the greater good in others or of a strong sense of belonging to a collective humanity and simply wanting to better connect with that humanity.

Why it's important (its benefits): Going through life believing that much weighs on your shoulders is very wearying. When we can sit in the "rest of the divine" or feel a sense of humanity's interconnectedness, strength, and shared positive intent, that yoke or burden feels lighter. It is shared. It's not all resting on me as an individual.

How to best put it into practice: Grow in spiritual disciplines. Make room for quietness. Practice gratitude. I recently read John Mark Comer's book, *The Ruthless Elimination of Hurry,* and was reminded again of the need—for me, at least—to have one day a week that looks very different from the others! I'm someone who often can fall into patterns of believing that if I let my guard down for one minute, don't work as hard one day, slack off too much, spend too much time reading a novel or hiking, or just doing nothing, that the world is going to crash and burn. Taking a day off from that weightiness reminds me that someone else has the omnipotence role covered!

Be a part of a faith community. Volunteer with others on a community need. And don't be surprised that if you are overly Type A like me, you might need a few extra hours of spiritual rest scattered throughout the week. Be open to whatever way that spiritual rest might appear!

Spiritual Rest 2-Year-Old Style

Until he was about ready for kindergarten, I cared for my little grandson, Primo, two days/a week. We'd go on grand adventure walks in our neighborhood, discovering new playgrounds, trails, and construction sites. We'd do puzzles, read, bake, play trains, color, and clean the house together. And we'd laugh—a lot!

It seemed like whenever Primo was over, something would have us in hilarious laughter, during which he'd remind me that "Primo is funny!"

I was recounting to a good friend one of Primo's and my uproarious incidents, so loudly uproarious that my husband—valiantly trying to work from home—had to come downstairs to see what all the noise and frivolity was about. Hearing the shared joy the incident produced, my friend, a non-religious but deeply spiritual woman, said to me, "It's like you babysit God." Then she corrected herself. "No, it's like God babysits you!"

Who knew that chasing after a very active grandchild could produce such profound rest, in this case, spiritual rest? You (and I) learn something new every day!

SIX TYPES OF REST WE OFTEN FORGET!

MENTAL - Schedule regular "brain breaks" and mindfulness, yoga or centered prayer to support the parasympathetic (rest) part of your autonomic nervous system.

EMOTIONAL - If you've been doing lots of giving or processing, an emotional time-out might be in order. Say "No" to people and things. Practice self-care.

SENSORY - Close your eyes (sleep mask), cover your ears (ear plugs) and take vacations from your devices to avoid sensory overload.

SOCIAL - Are there people or communities from which you need a rest? Is it possible to make more time for restorative relationships or spend more time alone?

CREATIVE - Determine if you need a break "for" or a break "from" creativity. Then pull out the paints and baking pans or up your joy by giving creativity a rest.

SPIRITUAL - Is it time to attend to what is beyond you and your routines? Connect with your sense of source and/or the common good in humanity.

Six Types of Rest

REST STOP

Time to take a break and digest information!

Take 10 minutes of calm to Rest with the following questions:

1. From where does it seem my major life stressors are coming?

2. What type of rest does it seem I most need?

Next, Stop for 10 minutes of quiet (sitting or slowly walking). Keep your mind as clear and open as possible, and just listen. Jot down any responses that may arise.

ROADWORK

Choose the option that most resonates with you. Note the option and your response in your *Trip Log*.

Option 1 – With what you believe to be your significant stressors and your most needed type of rest in mind, begin to get additionally curious about that rest. Approach it with the OCC exercise (Objectivity, Curiosity, and Compassion) and dig a bit deeper with these questions:

- Why do you focus your energy on these stressors during your day/week?

- Why does the type of rest you most need feel elusive or unattended to?

- What beliefs have you been taught or adopted about that type of rest?

- What are three ways you can begin to schedule and practice that type of rest?

Option 2 – If you've already done good exploratory work on your stressors and primary rest needs, begin to determine how much you need. At some point, we need some of all six types of rest, but for now, focusing on the area of most need, look at how much and how often you should incorporate that type of rest. How do you determine if you're getting the amount and frequency right? Notice what you are noticing.

Ask yourself:

- What am I noticing in my body, mind, and spirit?

- What most resonates with how I should respond to what I notice?

- What do I subsequently notice when I do or do not follow through on what I feel is best?

TRAVELLER ASSISTANCE – How to Grow a Good Habit (and weed a bad one!)

Ultimately, the journey toward metabolic health involves taking more actions supporting wellness and fewer negatively impacting wellness.

In essence, no behavior is neutral. It either moves you down the path toward illness or up the path toward wellness.

How to more simply increase actions that are wellness-producing!

While exploring Traffic Jams (wrong thinking) may still occasionally be needed, dealing with Road Blocks (wrong behavior) can be vastly easier when implementing these steps up the path to wellness rather than down the path to illness.

Adapting some of James Clear's counsel in his book, *Atomic Habits*, here's the starting place. To grow good habits, keep these four aspects in mind:

In Sight – The tools needed (running shoes, veggies, journal) to follow through on that habit should be in plain view.

Looks Good – Those tools must look appealing (quality footwear, fresh leafy greens, spanking new pages).

Super Simple – The habit must be straightforward rather than complex and detailed. (Head out the door, walk for 5 minutes, turn around, and return home.).

Feels Good – What you try to practice consistently must evoke positive responses (body, mind, or spirit joy).

Conversely, and now hopefully, understandably, you weed out a bad habit by paying attention to these four aspects:

Out of Sight – The foods that foster cravings and the TV remote are more challenging to access than your desired wellness tools and activities (Note that packing up all the sometimes foods—or those "almost never" ones—and keeping them in an out-of-the-way cupboard can be a good idea for many of us!).

Looks Bad – Any ultra-processed foods in the house are so far from your favorites that you'd be hard-pressed to look for them.

Super Hard – Unlocking your screen the times you've said you want to be screen-free requires a degree in software design.

Feels Bad – Without practicing guilt-tripping, remember why you're weeding out that bad habit. How does falling prey to it make you feel physically, emotionally, mentally, and spiritually?

SOUVENIR

Ultimately, what we are trying to accomplish in the practice of wise movement, sound sleep, and the following of good habits is to provide the tools for growth to a place of self-regulation. While self-regulation may be a new term to you, it is a practice with a long history of traditional use that has, as a by-product, the ability to increase energy.

Self-Regulation: An Energy Turbo-Charger!

We want to be able to notice what we are noticing in our bodies, be grateful for its messages, and learn the best ways to respond.

We want to *think* with our newer, more rational, and linear-thinking brain parts while *feeling* with our older, more emotional, and spontaneous-thinking emotional brain or limbic system.

Rest and Activity Prepare Us to Pay Attention

To remind you of this Leg of your Metabolic Health Roadmap, you can choose one item to purchase to support your desire to move and rest. You can buy brand new items online or in person or pick up items secondhand via a local thrift shop or virtual marketplace. Perhaps you will have a birthday or other celebratory occasion soon, or you can add the item to your "What do you want for Christmas?" list.

What is on Your Wishlist?

First, please review your notes, including your Rest Stop and RoadWork material, and see what resonates as a helpful reminder of your commitments to yourself. What will better allow you to establish habits fostering metabolic health and optimal wellness?
Options could be:
- A new pair of walking shoes or brightly colored shoelaces

- A better-quality pillow or beautiful new pillowcases

- Room-darkening shades or an eye mask

- A set of resistance bands or light weights

- Taking a creative mini-course (wedding cake baking, anyone?)

Then, prepare for a rested state that will set the stage for our deep dive, next Leg, into more understanding of and support tools for a foundational metabolic wellness topic—self-regulation.

Chapter Sixteen

LEG 5 - Manage Stress for Metabolic Health

SUMMARY – Travel Size Version

Where in this Leg, You'll Discover that Everyone Experiences Stress and Not all Stress is Necessarily Bad for You.

However, what is vital to metabolic health and optimal wellness is the growth in stress management understanding and skills!

Diagnostic #4 - Paying Attention to Paradigms

For Leg 5, your Diagnostic is to reflect on the SEE and SHIFT section under each paradigm and note which paradigm resonates most obviously as the one you will work on in your Rest Stop and RoadWork exercises.

Attitude: Seeing and Shifting Paradigms

Thus far, we've covered B-Body Type, A-Activity, N-good Night's sleep, C-Clean water, and E-Eat for health in our metabolic BALANCE acronym. In this Leg, we look at the first A-Attitude and L-Laughter and play.

For attitude, it can be easy to say, "Attitude is everything; might as well choose a good one!" The challenge is it's not always easy to change your attitude and choose a good one. That's why we'll look at the paradigms—biases, and beliefs—that underlie the attitudes so real and sustainable change becomes possible.

The Shift Above All Shifts!

Here, you'll discover what may be the most straightforward and most powerful step to increased energy and optimal wellness: gratitude! I'll give you many benefits and practical steps to set thankfulness in place!

Laughter and Play

Who knew the massive wellness benefits of fitting more laughter and play into one's life? This section is where the expenditure of time and labor resources results in a massive Net Energy Gain! It even includes a tasty recipe to enjoy during a stress-busting movie or games night.

Habit Hitching

In the last Leg, we looked at Seed Habits—how to grow good ones and weed out bad ones. Here, I'll give you a few principles on efficiently and sustainably implementing those habits even with a very full schedule.

It's the Breath in Your Lungs

Regular inhales and exhales of breath are essential for life, and how we monitor and regulate that breathing can go a long way to helping manage stress. As this Leg's Souvenir, I'll give you some breathwork options.

Chapter Seventeen

LEG 5 - Manage Stress: Getting Started

"Midlife is when the universe gently places her hand upon your shoulders, pulls you close, and whispers in your ear: I'm not screwing around. All of this pretending and performing—these coping mechanisms that you've developed to protect yourself from feeling inadequate and getting hurt—has to go."

Brené Brown

W hile immediate energy trumps everything and is why we start the metabolic health journey with eating well for your body type, eventually having an endless supply of that energy will require digging a little deeper. To paraphrase Brené Brown's words, it is time to stop with the mind games and get real, not only with your food intake but with how you think and feel.

Managing stress and, therefore, freeing up the copious amounts of energy that not managing stress takes is the ultimate wellness pairing with the first few Legs' eating well, moving well, and sleeping well!

And, as with the topic of most Legs, the relationship between stress and metabolic health is complex and deeply intertwined. The bonus? Managing one can substantially improve the other!

In what ways?

Let's start with the way improved metabolic health enhances stress management outcomes:

Better balanced hormones - As with food intake, exercise, and sleep, improving metabolic health has positive ripple effects on our hormones, particularly stress-related hormones like cortisol, epinephrine, and norepinephrine.

Increased energy - When metabolic health is improved, along with a more efficient and effective conversion of food to cellular energy, there is typically an uptick in overall physical energy. And that, in turn, improves resilience and ability to cope with stress.

Decreased systemic inflammation - Chronic inflammation can exacerbate our body's stress response and contribute to mood disorders such as anxiety and depression. Because improved metabolic health can reduce inflammation, there is also often a corresponding ability to better manage stress.

And how can better stress management positively impact metabolic health? Let's look at those pathways as well:

Decreased risk of metabolic syndrome - Chronic stress contributes to the expression of various ailments, including increased blood pressure, high blood sugar levels, excess visceral fat, and poor cholesterol levels. Better stress management can reduce some of those risk factors.

Improved insulin sensitivity - When you better manage stress, you can improve insulin sensitivity. Chronic stress and the hormones produced by that stress can make the body's cells less responsive to insulin.

Reduced visceral fat - One critical component of sound metabolic health is controlling abdominal fat levels. Visceral fat levels are mainly influenced by cortisol. Reducing stress, therefore, can directly impact fat accumulation around internal organs.

When you enhance any aspect of metabolic health or stress management, you have the potential to foster improvement in the other, creating, as it were, a cycle of increasing health benefits. So, where are you in that cycle?

As usual, we'll start with a simple diagnostic check-up.

Diagnostic #4 – Key Paradigm to See and Shift

This Leg's Diagnostic is easy. It requires no extra effort besides reading the material in the Information Centre and paying attention to which of the five paradigms we'll cover resonates as the key one you want to work on.

Be aware, as was the case with me and many of my clients and workshop participants, that all five paradigms may cause bells to ring and lights to flash in your brain as "pick me" paradigms. If so, you will eventually want to examine them all more deeply.

But, for starters, pick just one! That paradigm will be the focus of this Leg's Rest Stop and RoadWork exercises.

Chapter Eighteen

LEG 5 - Attitude - Seeing and Shifting Paradigms

"Something will control the way you move forward physically, emotionally, and spiritually . . . it might as well be you!"

Brenda Wollenberg

INFORMATION CENTRE

In the quest for metabolic health, an often-overlooked factor is our attitude or emotions.

With exciting discoveries in various fields, including quantum physics, neuroscience, epigenetics, and psychology, we are uncovering significant links between our beliefs and feelings and how our lives unfold.

In *Becoming Supernatural*, author Dr. Joe Dispenza describes emotions as:

> *"the chemical consequences (or feedback) of past experiences ... as our senses record incoming information from the environment, clusters of neurons organize into networks. When they freeze into a pattern, the brain makes a chemical that is then sent throughout the body. That chemical is called an emotion."*

Our body's creation of and subsequent responses to those chemicals—or, as we typically refer to them, those emotions—can lock us into patterns of less-than-helpful behavior.

Dr. Dispenza says:

> *"Because of our large brains, human beings can think about their problems, relive past events, or even forecast future worst-case situations and thus turn on the cascade of stress chemicals by thought alone. We can knock our brains out of normal physiology just by thinking about an all-too-familiar past or trying to control an unpredictable future."*

HOW EMOTIONS ARE MADE

Our senses record incoming information from our environment.	Clusters of neurons organize into networks and then freeze into a pattern.	The brain makes a chemical that is sent throughout the body. That chemical is called an emotion.

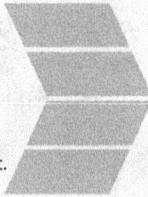

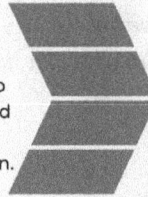

Per Dr. Joe Dispenza in *Becoming Supernatural*

How Emotions Are Made

Additionally, in new research on trauma, doctors and scientists are finding that suffering, pain, and distress can set the stage for ongoing survival tactics, even when those tactics may not be needed in a current situation. So, while we can be collectively thankful for that large brain, it is in our best interests to realize that it comes with some survival-mode "software" that we need to address to manage stress well and have our body|mind|spirit thrive.

MANAGING "SURVIVAL MODE" SOFTWARE

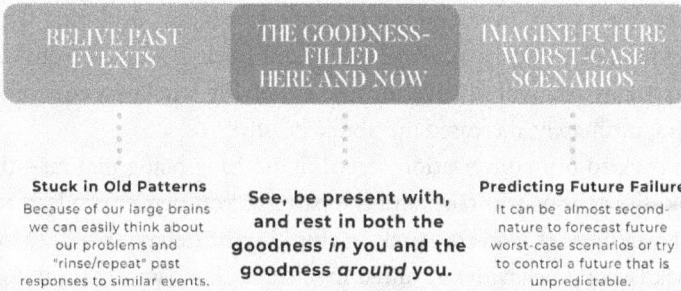

RELIVE PAST EVENTS	THE GOODNESS-FILLED HERE AND NOW	IMAGINE FUTURE WORST-CASE SCENARIOS
Stuck in Old Patterns Because of our large brains we can easily think about our problems and "rinse/repeat" past responses to similar events.	**See, be present with, and rest in both the goodness *in* you and the goodness *around* you.**	**Predicting Future Failure** It can be almost second-nature to forecast future worst-case scenarios or try to control a future that is unpredictable.

Per Dr. Joe Dispenza in *Becoming Supernatural*

Managing "Survival Mode" Software

The Internal Forces that Motivate Us

Fortunately, along with scientific advances in research on the connections between physical, emotional, mental, and spiritual health, better ways of understanding the internal forces that motivate us are also being developed. We are seeing a broader grasp of crucial factors needed in healthy child development and the not-yet-sufficient but at least wider availability of trauma-informed counseling and support for people of all ages. There is growing awareness of the importance of sound mental health, how mental health can be negatively impacted, and the various complementary ways to address those challenges.

Traumatic-Stress Support

And, before we begin looking at Attitude, please note that should anything in this Leg (or any other Leg, for that matter) reveal the need for more in-depth inner exploration and a more complex set of understanding and resources, seek professional help.

While this Leg covers a helpful set of See and Shift tools for revealing and circumventing or dissolving blocks, paradigms, or biases that might currently be challenging you physically, emotionally, or spiritually, it is not a substitute for counseling or therapy. Should that be a need, seek the support of a trauma-informed counselor or therapist who has an array of tools at their disposal (EMDR, somatic experiencing, internal family systems therapy).

Origins of Paradigms (You need to see them before you can shift them!)

In this Leg, we'll cover five common paradigms or biases, exploring which will allow you to gain *energy* by understanding and freeing yourself from *stuckness*. How you might ask, will discovering and dissolving stuckness equate to more energy and, ultimately, increased metabolic health?

Think back to our conversation regarding nothing being neutral—the ways you think, the actions you take, and the patterns you perpetuate lead to either illness or wellness. If you are stuck in thinking or behavior—thwarted by a Roadblock (wrong behavior) or mired in a Traffic Jam (wrong thinking)—it is not a neutral experience. You are being prevented from moving forward toward increased wellness.

As you explore these five paradigms—the names and concepts that I initially encountered in a tiny but powerful book by Brian McLaren called *Why Don't They Get It? Overcoming Bias in Others (and yourself)*—and grow in your ability to recognize and circumvent them, you'll spend less downtime in the "shop" and more time on the open road, heading toward your wellness destination!

But first, before we start tackling ways to examine these perhaps all-too-familiar paradigms and determine if adhering to them is in our best interest . . .

What Exactly is a Paradigm, and Where Do They Come From?

Paradigms can also be described as biases or world views. They are:

- A model – A typical example of something

- A framework – Unwritten rules that direct actions

- A set of concepts – A manner of looking at something

- A thought pattern – A basic assumption or way of thinking

Understand that the concept of a paradigm itself is neutral. Like the word "value" or "guideline," it simply describes a structure or foundation through which we interpret, define and engage in the world.

Paradigms develop in a variety of ways but primarily through:

- Patterning – Thoughts, phrases, and beliefs we repeat

- Programming – Things others have repeatedly said or done to us

- Habits – The culmination of patterning and programming

We Think and Behave the Way We Do Because of Our Paradigms

Everyone has paradigms that impact their unique way of seeing the world. The ways we interpret an event (our boss letting a co-worker go) or the meanings we ascribe to a statement someone makes (our partner asking if we remembered to pick up eggs for dinner) are at least, in part, because of the paradigms we hold.

But Where Do Paradigms REALLY Come From?

For this, we need a mini-science lesson and a look back in history. Way back!

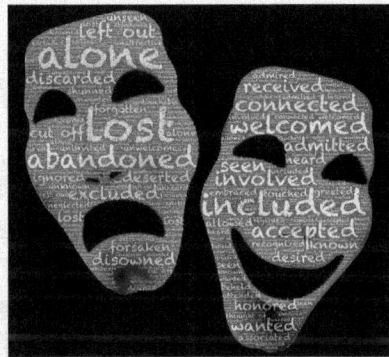

How to Describe Them

- A model - a typical example
- A framework - unwritten rules
- A set of concepts - a manner of looking at something
- A thought pattern - a basic assumption

How They Develop

- Patterning - things we repeat
- Programming - things others have said/done to us
- Habits - the culmination of patterning and programming

Paradigms

Emotional Brain

The emotional brain (also called the reptilian or limbic brain) is the oldest part of our brain. It has two guiding—largely subconscious—principles by which it operates:

- Self-protection – It responds quickly to provide safety

- Self-interest – It responds quickly to promote that which will most benefit us

This part of our brain has us jump over a nearby hedge when we see a car being driven erratically toward us as we're out on a walk. The rational part of our brain would have us calculating perceived speed and likely travel distances over a specific time. Our emotional brain has us quickly leap to safety before our rational brain gets even part-way through the mathematical calculation.

Rational Brain

The rational or cognitive part of our brain is the newest and is mainly concerned with the world around us. This part works to understand how people and things function. It determines how to set goals and meet those goals. Time management and scheduling our day are all aspects of rational or cognitive functioning.

Self-Regulation: The Best of Both Worlds

While the actions of the emotional brain can, at times, contribute to feelings of embarrassment or confusion (the reckless driver corrected their direction and speed; all we got for our leap to "safety" was a sprained ankle and a tear in our new jeans), we are here today because of physically life-sustaining—survival of the fittest—paradigms.

The key to stress management wellness is to learn how to have each part of the brain better recognize and pay attention to the other's beneficial skill set—in a hyphenated word, self-regulation.

The rational brain can merrily go on its way, thinking in straight lines, planning linearly, and focusing on staying calm, relaxed, and collected. It can easily downplay, ignore or not even consciously be aware of messages the emotional brain is sending ("I said jump, dammit!!").

Likewise, the emotional brain, too, can be highly single-minded. It acts very quickly. And, by the very nature of its design, it is not very rational! The emotional brain is why we have had to come up with—and often use—apologies such as: "Sorry about that; I spoke/behaved/acted without thinking!"

According to Dr. Bessel van der Kolk's explanation in his excellent and highly recommended book, *The Body Keeps the Score*, the old part of our brain is the part that controls everything a baby can generally automatically do when born: " *eat, sleep, wake up, breathe, feel temperature, hunger, wetness, and pain and rid the body of toxins by urinating and defecating.* "

Each time you get caught up in a wellness Traffic Jam (wrong thinking) that can be identified as dealing with any of those "baby can do" comfort aspects of our being—safety, threat, hunger, fatigue, desire, longing, excitement, pleasure and pain—get curious about what lies beneath that Traffic Jam. As you compassionately ask questions and evaluate root causes, self-protection or self-interest are likely at play. It is also possible that self-protection or self-interest is not warranted in the current situation.

In the next section of this Leg and the following Leg, we'll dig a little deeper into ways to self-regulate, including the use of the BALANCE "L" of Laughter and play, but for now, as we go through the five primary paradigms that most of us contend with, see which of the recommended tools resonate as the one that will help you shift your wellness thinking and eventually, therefore, your wellness behavior. That, in turn, will free up time and labor resources and increase the odds of you improving metabolic health.

Keys to Paradigm Shift

As we explore managing stress by identifying and, if necessary, shifting paradigms, remember that paradigms are essential. They are shortcuts that help us easily define what we see, hear, and feel and let us know how to proceed. Without paradigms, we would constantly struggle to figure out our next step and best make plans to move forward.

As you examine each paradigm, be gracious and kind to yourself and probably extend a bit of gratitude to your emotional brain for saving your butt as many times as it has! However, you will likely see a few paradigms you no longer want to hold. Or you want to hold them differently.

Perhaps they aren't serving you well or at all anymore. You may realize you want to see and think somewhat—or even wholly—differently. You may decide that, in fact, some of these paradigms have been overprotecting you or falsely attending to your best interests.

Any of those options would be excellent observations. The good news is that you can change how you think!

Change the Way You Think

The key to a paradigm shift centers on these two factors:

1. **Holding your paradigms loosely:** keep an open mind about your usual way of being and doing.

2. **Being open to new information:** when you reform or replace your thinking, you become a new person.

Instead of being stuck in old thought patterns and behaviors, be willing to think about things differently. Be open, expand, consider, and be willing to be wrong.

It takes great courage and effort to see and shift paradigms. Holding paradigms that no longer effectively move us up the road to optimal wellness also takes tremendous effort. You might as well use those time and labor resources to produce a larger Energy Net Gain and enhanced overall health!

Now, on to five common paradigms, you'll want to learn how to SEE and, perhaps, SHIFT.

#1 Comfort Paradigm

In short, this is the paradigm where we prefer not to disturb our comfort or complacency!

A properly functioning emotional brain is adept at conserving and protecting our emotional, physical, and mental energy. It doesn't want to take on any more than it already handles.

Witness the concept of "compassion fatigue." When we are inundated with ongoing news stories or a flooding of our social media accounts with words and scenes of a tragic event, it eventually becomes too much. We change the channel to a sitcom or power down our device and go to bed.

See It
- Routine rules – You find that spontaneity has gone the way of the dodo bird, and you like the familiar to the extreme (You eat the same two veggies every day. AKA you're in a rut!).

- You don't rock the boat – If an idea or response percolates that might require moving outside your comfort zone, it immediately gets suppressed. (You think about turning off the TV and getting to bed an hour earlier . . . and immediately talk yourself out of it!)

Shift It
- Mix it up – Planfully incorporate new activities into your life. Follow different people on Instagram. Read new authors. Listen to new music. Try one new vegetable each week!

- Allow for a detour – When that new or different idea or response arises, follow it up. Be willing to explore something atypical, even if it makes you nervous. Next time the "turn off the TV an hour early" message floats through your brain, compromise and start with 15-30 minutes earlier.

#2. Confirmation Paradigm

With Confirmation Paradigms, we judge new ideas based on the ease with which they fit in and confirm the only standard we have. That standard is based on:

- Old ideas

- Old information

- Currently trusted authorities

This is the most common bias, and it's a strong one! Again, it is our emotional brain's way of conserving energy, this time intellectual energy. We all have filters through which we run new information. Does this or does this not fit with what I already know? Does this puzzle piece of new knowledge fit with the old?

This filtering does not necessarily come from a desire to be bad-mannered or unenlightened; it simply corresponds with our emotional brain's attempt at efficiency.

Evaluating something new thoroughly takes time and energy. When protecting those resources, accepting or rejecting something based on what most closely aligns with what we already think is more manageable.

See It

- Do a one-year review – Look back one year, or even one month, and review your life. Does it look the same or different? Are you taking new walking paths? Are you meeting new friends?

- Do you behave like your parents? – We all carry forward traits from our family of origin. Some of those traits are wonderful; some not so much. Are you doing things as your mom or dad did because they are valuable practices or because they are long-held and unchallenged beliefs?

Shift It

- Do a one-year forward Gratitude Review. Look ahead one year or even one month, and review your life. What will you be thankful you spent time on during that year or month? What fruits of your effort will produce the most gratefulness when you do the review? Incorporate more of those activities. Use your imagination! Creativity is always helpful, particularly with this paradigm.

- I AM statements – Create a list of five I AM statements (I am loved. I am persevering. I am wise. I am worthy. I am confident.) and recite the statements daily. I AM statements are deeply powerful!

○ However, I AM statements need to be set on a foundation of hope and possibility. Simply making statements in which you have not one iota of faith won't work. If you have difficulty believing your I AM statements, make them easier to believe (I am kind. I have potential.). Pay particular attention to the gratitude information in this Leg's Traveller Assistance section. Gratitude helps create an entirely different internal thought terrain and is an excellent place to begin with transformational body|mind|spirit work.

#3. Community Paradigm

The truth is that people mainly change their minds when the pain of not changing surpasses the pain of changing. And that change is complicated when their surrounding community doesn't, can't, or won't see a need for it.

Peer pressure is genuine. What will friends think if I adopt this line of reasoning or action? Will co-workers still respect/like/value me if they know I feel differently than they do about x, y, or z?

We pretty well all like to belong (again, hard-wired—part of a "safety in numbers" emotional brain response), and almost no one longs for rejection. What others THINK is a big deal. And we tend to think more effortlessly when aligned with the thoughts of those around us. Swimming upstream "belief-wise" takes a lot of emotional and mental work!

See It
- Go with the flow – Is your primary method of operation to check the pulse of those surrounding you and then to vote, order, listen, attend, watch, dress, and vacation the way they do?

- Rinse and repeat – With the backing of your community, do you keep attempting things or starting things over, but you don't achieve the results you were hoping for?

Shift It
- Take a stand – While not intentionally trying to be contrary, consider internal nudges to think or act differently. Do your research. Come to some of your own conclusions.

- Get outside input – Seek out those with a different worldview than those you generally hang out with. Hire a coach. Work with a nutritionist.

#4. Complexity Paradigm

Our brains prefer a simple falsehood (2 + 4 = 7) to a complex truth.

We've been talking about how paradigms help conserve physical and emotional energy. They are also super good at preserving our intellectual energy. With complex issues, our emotional brain shuts the door to helpful analysis before the topic can introduce itself. That's because the brain has a lot on the go and can only juggle so many pressing concerns. The emotional brain automatically says "No!" to allowing the rational brain the time it needs for in-depth review.

See It

- A *Cole's Notes* life – You live a *Reader's Digest Condensed Book* of everything: literature, food, relationships, passions, and dreams. Your wellness practice only scratches the surface of what is available to understand and adopt. You realize you are not going deep in any areas and are not using your brain power to wisely examine how you are "Being" and what you are "Doing."

- Easy way out – You are not prepared to spend the resources (time, energy, or money) getting to a fuller, more complex understanding of a topic. The latest book on fitness research does not make your "must-read" list.

Shift It

- KISS as a starting point – Implement the *Keep it Simple, Silly* principle only where appropriate. There is a place for a 1500-word article or a 90-minute workshop. But information in bullet form is a starting point. It is meant to whet your appetite and not to be the whole or complete answer.

- You get what you pay for – Investing additional time and energy in learning produces a more extensive, often more robust, and nuanced truth. Start simply, but invite yourself to and reward yourself for greater depth.

#5. Confidence Paradigm

We are attracted to confidence, even if it is false. We often prefer the bold lie to the hesitant truth.

Those two statements don't say much about our innate powers of discernment, but remember, we are wired for survival. We look for boldness, a strong leader, and a fast leader (to protect us from a circling ambush of saber-toothed tigers!). We don't often listen to a humble, quiet voice, which can be problematic.

Remember the classic childhood storybook with the resultant "The Emperor has No Clothes" syndrome. If we only follow the lead of the noisiest or "highest" authority, we can easily be manipulated.

See It

- Pull of the familiar – If you are still listening only to the loud and flashy voices of your childhood or young adulthood, you may have been lulled into "falsehood."

- Lack of due diligence – Confident voices can sweep us up in a facade of truth and keep us from appropriate examination and evaluation.

Shift It

- Grow your confidence – List your accomplishments and things you do well. Stand up for yourself and your beliefs. Practice speaking your truth clearly and confidently.

- Follow through in evaluation and listening! Get good at discerning BS (even, and maybe especially, if it is spoken boldly, showily, and loudly) and recognizing truth (even if it comes across quietly and haltingly).

FIVE PRIMARY PARADIGMS

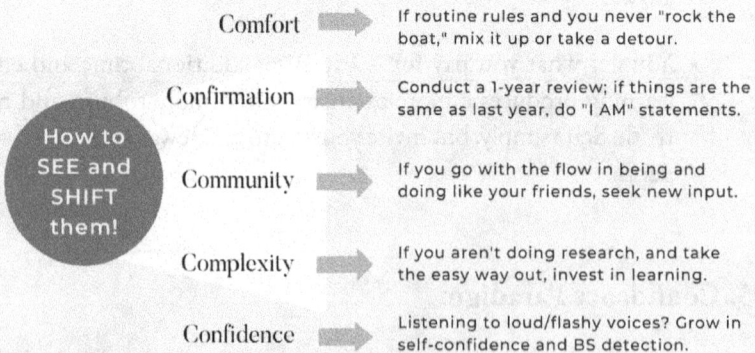

	Comfort ➡	If routine rules and you never "rock the boat," mix it up or take a detour.
	Confirmation ➡	Conduct a 1-year review; if things are the same as last year, do "I AM" statements.
How to SEE and SHIFT them!	Community ➡	If you go with the flow in being and doing like your friends, seek new input.
	Complexity ➡	If you aren't doing research, and take the easy way out, invest in learning.
	Confidence ➡	Listening to loud/flashy voices? Grow in self-confidence and BS detection.

Five Primary Paradigms

A Personal Paradigm-Busting Story

Like most of us, I grew up with strong paradigms. Some were decent and are ones I've kept to this day:

- Family matters

- Suppers should be eaten together

- Celebrate the little things

But I also found myself with many self-protective and self-promoting paradigms that, as an adult, were NOT serving me well. Ones like:

- Life is hard

- Work before play

- People will let you down

- Keep your guard up

All of these contributed to me being a fairly skeptical, nose-to-the-grindstone, not going to win any "fun person of the year" awards, and an ulcer-producing workaholic. Much of my vocabulary revolved around words like *not, no, won't,* and *but.*

Over time, I realized the foundational underpinnings of much of my behavior and personality (took time to SEE them) were no longer principles I believed or wanted to walk out (desired to SHIFT them). I wanted to be a more joyful, less negative, more spontaneous, and more open-to-goodness person. And I began taking steps to move forward on that wellness/stress management journey.

- I ate more real food (for my body type) and WAY less sugar.

- I found a physical activity I enjoyed doing and did it regularly.

- I created a sleep routine and adjusted it until it worked.

- I upped my thankfulness (became grateful not necessarily "for" everything but "in" everything).

After a year of practicing these principles, I overheard a woman say, "You are the most positive person I have ever met!" I turned around to see to whom the statement was being directed and, at that moment, realized that, miraculously, it was being spoken to me!

I instantly became sold on paradigm-busting for life!

REST STOP

Time to take a break and digest information!

Take 10 minutes of calm to Rest with the following questions:

1. Which of the five presented paradigms most resonated as something for you to explore?

2. What do you SEE of its evidence in your life? Are there aspects of that paradigm that you would like to SHIFT?

Next, Stop for 10 minutes of quiet (sitting or slowly walking). Keep your mind as clear and open as possible, and just listen. Jot down any responses that may arise.

ROADWORK

Choose the option that most resonates with you. Note the option and your response in your *Trip Log*.

Often, we think of exercises such as examining biases and paradigms like these as "extra" or "fluff" work. We'll get to it at some point, but it's not a top priority; it doesn't seem highly relevant to something as physical and tangible as increasing energy, and the time and labor resources required for introspection seem unlikely to produce a large Energy Net Gain.

I used to think that.

My thinking, however, could not have been further from the truth. Indeed, it was seeing and shifting this Leg's and other biases and beliefs that were foundational to how I corrected my underactive thyroid, to how I found the right body size for me and pretty much stayed there, to how my brain got clearer, to how I—most days now—have energy to burn, to how I fight hard for authenticity and depth in relationships, and to how I have a more genuine sense of spiritual calmness and grounding.

Digging deeper into those topics is for another Leg (or, realistically, another book!). But those behaviors wouldn't have happened without some simple and regular (and often repetitive!) shifting of the types of paradigms found in this Leg.

Option 1 – Dig a little deeper into the paradigm you found most resonating in this Leg's Rest Stop:

- From where do you think it originated?

- What part of your "be, do, have, and give" Faith Goals does that paradigm no longer serve?

- Which of the SHIFT recommendations listed under each Paradigm can you use to move on from that paradigm?

- How will shifting that paradigm make it easier to follow through on your wellness Action Goals?

- Where might those recommendations come in handy on your journey to wellness?

Option 2 – Consider whether you are a grateful person. Ask yourself:

- Do I believe I'm a self-made person, or am I grateful for the input of others and source?

- Does "Thank you!" roll often from my lips?

- Do I believe that goodness runs after me (and often catches up) or that things generally don't work out in my favor?

- What methods can I use to incorporate more gratitude into my life? (Suggestions would be to start a gratitude journal, begin each day verbally listing three things for which you are most grateful, or express specific thankfulness to two people—whether in person or by other means—each day.)

- How will increasing gratitude in my life make it easier to follow through on the Action Goals I say are important to me?

TRAVELLER ASSISTANCE – The Power of Gratitude

What if there was a simple, potent step to facilitate the shift from internal confusion, fatigue, and irritation to joy, endless energy, and overall wellness?

Well, guess what . . . there is. Gratitude.

Gratitude: The Strong and Mighty Step that Starts the Shift

Whether framed religiously, philosophically, or intellectually, the human condition is such that we are profoundly dependent on others. We should be grateful for that dependence on others and on whatever links us to the beyond. (On days I doubt this, I ask my body, mind, and spirit, "Seriously, do we really want me to be our sole resource?")

Looking for reasons to incorporate more thanksgiving into your life?

- **Gratitude makes us fully human:** And it is likely an evolutionarily beneficial trait. Think about how gratitude helps you initiate and foster relationships, and then consider that in terms of alliances and survival!

- **Feeling grateful is good for you:** A grateful attitude produces happiness, satisfaction with life, hope, and a sense of meaning. It can also reduce anxiety and depression.

- **Expressions of gratitude can be personalized to suit you:** Write gratitude in a diary or journal, express it verbally as daily reminders or affirmations, dance, or otherwise express your gratitude through movement.

- **For a double bonus, practice quiet gratitude:** Intentional silent reflection on what you are thankful for produces optimism and increased life satisfaction. It also makes room for new awareness and growth to arise!

We only move on to increased understanding with stillness, quietness, and reflection. Gratitude sets the stage for that!

> *"Gratitude is the truest approach to life.*
> *We did not create or fashion ourselves.*
> *We did not birth ourselves.*
> *Life is about giving, receiving, and repaying.*
> *We are receptive beings, dependent on the help of others,*
> *on their gifts and their kindness."*

Robert Emmons, Psychologist, University of California, Davis

GRATITUDE

The strong and mighty step that starts the shift!

Gratitude Makes Us Fully Human

Likely an evolutionary beneficial trait, gratitude helps initiate and foster relationships.

Feeling Grateful is Good for You

A grateful attitude produces happiness, satisfaction with life, hope, and a sense of meaning.

Gratitude is Universal

We are born, survive off the generosity of others, and then pass on. Gratitude is a principle of life.

Personalize Your Gratitude

Write out gratitude, express gratitude verbally or express your gratitude through movement.

Practice Gratitude Quietly

In addition, pair gratitude with silent reflection. It produces optimism and makes room for growth.

Gratitude

Chapter Nineteen

LEG 5 - Laughter and Play

"I have always felt that laughter in the face of reality is probably the finest sound there is and will last until the day when the game is called on account of darkness. In this world, a good time to laugh is any time you can."

Linda Ellerbee, American Journalist

Information Centre

How much does laughter and play contribute to managing stress and ultimately to optimal energy and health? Well, enough that we've been hearing about it, even anecdotally, for almost 500 years.

Besides rescuing you from being stuck in a *same old, same old* paradigm pattern or luring you to break from a boring workout routine to watch a comedy at your local theatre—while munching down liberally buttered popcorn—laughter and play adds an interesting element when planning your Action and even your Faith Goals. It is essential to schedule some fun—like that night at the movies or an afternoon of bocce at the park—for successful results when setting real goals to accomplish real health.

Laughter for Release of Excess Stored Body Fat

On a side note, for readers looking to release excess stored fat, the good news is research that 10-15 minutes of knee-slapping belly laughs can burn up to 50 calories worth of energy, similar to energy burned during a brisk walk.

As mentioned in my book *Overweight Kids in a Toothpick World*, research from a professor at Stanford University, William Fry, has determined that 20 seconds of hearty laughter is comparable to three minutes of arduous rowing. What is even more interesting, however, particularly in the Manage Stress for Metabolic Health Leg, is that when it comes to laughter and play, laughter is a vital force that can lessen the effects of stress on the body.

Our Love/Hate Relationship with Cortisol

Cortisol, a well-utilized hormone in the emotional brain tool kit, is the hormone that allows the body to react efficiently in times of danger, with a fight, flight, or freeze response that is helpful under specific circumstances. However, due to excess daily stress from strict deadlines at work, unbearable traffic, or watching your kid challenge gravity from high up on the playground monkey bars, cortisol levels can reach unnecessary, high, or fluctuating (at the wrong times of the day) levels in the body.

Because of the wide range of stress we're currently surrounded by, stress can become chronic. Even at low levels, this relentlessly ongoing stress becomes a serious challenge when trying to obtain increased energy and optimal wellness, as high cortisol levels were never meant to be the norm.

Are you concerned that high or erratic cortisol levels could be an issue? Here are a few signs of cortisol imbalance:

- Food cravings

- Storage of visceral fat (fat surrounding abdominal organs)

- Diabetes

- Insomnia

Knowing that laughter potently lowers cortisol levels, you can see how it could be a helpful tool on your metabolic health journey. Here are two tools to incorporate fun into your Action Goals, keep you motivated, and assist in gaining the results you are looking for.

Two Key Ways to Use Laughter and Play for Managing Stress

Make Room for Play

Time to get a little "immature" please!

- **Be childlike** – Plan board game nights with friends or a family dance session.

- **Be spontaneous** – Try something new—a recipe, a different fitness class at your community center, Hawaiian shirt day, or a Master Chef cook-off in your kitchen.

- **Be creative** – Make cooking a team effort and have your partner or child choose, from a few options, some of the foods for dinner, or create a cooking playlist to listen to during food prep.

- **Be a play promoter** – Promoting play as a parent, partner, or friend teaches the importance of regular fun and play to those with whom you are in a relationship.

Use Positive and Playful Communication

Language is a powerful tool in determining what we think of ourselves. Self-communication around essential concepts such as acceptance, recognition of unconditional love, and belief in innate worthiness are key aspects in managing stress.

- **Language re-frames** – Rather than exclaiming, "I want to be skinny," choose language that builds you up: "I want to be comfortable in my body" or "I want to reach my best-for-me body size." Rather than proclaiming, "I'm on a diet," try "I am changing to a health-supporting lifestyle," which backs the choice to adopt healthier long-term action steps rather than a temporary fix found in following a "diet."

- **The "yet" word** – Consider, as well, the playful use of the word "yet." I haven't figured out the best way to fall asleep quickly . . . yet. I haven't made it out for my walk, 5 out of 7 days . . . yet. This slight addition shows intent, doesn't invalidate your less-than-exact accomplishments, and can prevent discouragement.

While being playful and choosing positive communication can seem a step or two removed from stress management, both practices are conscious decisions to choose proactive change. Knowing where you are headed (Faith Goals) and implementing concrete steps (Action Goals) to reach that destination are very effective stress management tools.

Who knew having fun was crucial to a sustainable wellness plan?

A Tasty Recipe for a Laughter and Play Night

Keep your goals fun and exciting, and when you schedule one of those game or movie nights, enjoy this tasty, stress-busting Nibbles recipe, too!

It is adapted from a recipe created by one of my favorite people, my wonderful step-mom, Joyce.

Ingredients:

6 cups popped non-GMO popcorn
1 cup natural sesame cracker strips
1 cup natural pretzel sticks
1 ½ cups natural "O" cereal
2 cups natural "wheat square" cereal
1 cup natural cheese crackers
2 cups mixed nuts (raw, unsalted)

Directions:

In a small saucepan, combine, stirring until butter melts:
¾ cup butter (or ½ butter, ½ olive oil)
1½ tsp. Spike or Herbamare seasoning
½ tsp. celery salt
10 drops Tabasco sauce
1 tsp. onion powder
1 tsp. garlic powder

Pour the butter mixture over the dry ingredients, place the nibbles in a large roasting pan, and bake at 250 degrees for 1 hour, stirring frequently. Allow to cool completely. Serve.

REST STOP

Time to take a break and digest information!

Take 10 minutes of calm to Rest with the following questions:

1. When do I play? And in what way?

2. What do I believe about taking time for play?

Next, Stop for 10 minutes of quiet (sitting or slowly walking). Keep your mind as clear and open as possible, and just listen. Jot down any responses that may arise.

ROADWORK

Choose the option that most resonates with you. Note the option and your response in your *Trip Log*.

As adults, we often associate laughter and play with childhood. Our communication usually takes a sombre note as we "mature."

Today's RoadWork examines ways to restore lightness and joy because those two characteristics almost always partner with improved metabolic health.

Option 1 – Where can you begin incorporating more play into your life?

- Do you have an old hobby you can revive?

- Is there a sport you used to play that you can begin again?

- What type of creativity resides inside of you? Dance? Crafting? Cookie decorating? Songwriting? Schedule time to nurture that creativity.

- If you lack inspiration for incorporating more play, borrow—with permission—a young child, roughly 3-5 years of age. Follow them around for a day. Do what they do. Explore what they explore. Laugh and be silly when they laugh and be silly. Inspiration should arise. If not, rinse and repeat until it does.

Option 2 – Does your self-talk need a tune-up?

- Do you feel that maturity = solemness in how you talk to yourself?

- Do you often self-correct or berate yourself?

- Do you believe you have a solid core of intrinsic value, or does that value seem dependent on your behavior or accomplishments?

- Consider talking to yourself with the kindness, compassion, and expectation for perfection you would have with a 5-year-old you love and care about.

- Begin practicing using the "yet" word discussed above under Language Re-frames.

TRAVELLER ASSISTANCE – Habit Hitching

Habit hitching is a simple but powerful three-step method for following through on what you say is important to you. Inspired by James Clear's super helpful book *Atomic Habits*, habit hitching uses practices you already do well as a framework for adding new helpful behaviors to your wellness routine.

When you decide on Action Goals, you'd like to begin to implement (hopefully, starting with one new goal in each of the seven areas of BALANCE), write them in your *Trip Log* and then execute the three following steps to begin incorporating your Action Goals for life successfully:

1. **Clearly define your Action Goal.** Later, you'll have more complex Action Goals; perhaps you'll want to run a ½ marathon one day and need an extensive series of more in-depth Action Goals. But to begin with, the goal should be small (take 2-5 minutes to complete), simple (one action), sensible (convenient), and sustainable (trackable). For example, a goal of five minutes of seated quiet contemplation five evenings a week.

2. **Find an action you already do consistently well.** You may be excellent at brushing and flossing your teeth each night. You never miss a day and are motivated to continue the practice forever because your dental hygienist praises you regularly!

3. **Hitch the new action you'd like to establish as a habit to your already-established habit.** After brushing and flossing, move to a comfortable chair in the next room, set your timer for five minutes, shut your eyes, and begin your practice of quiet contemplation. That's it! Your chances of continuing your new action have increased significantly by hitching it to a habit you already regularly and naturally practice.

Note that initially, you may need reminders to hitch the new action to the habitual action. After all, your habit used to end with a rinse and spit!

Put a sticky note on your bathroom mirror or tack a bright red bow to your contemplation chair. Eventually, however, your habit of hitching will "take," and the new action will feel as comfortable, regular, and easy to complete as the old habit!

SOUVENIR

One of the simplest and most effective ways to manage stress is with specific breathing patterns that support the parasympathetic side of our autonomic nervous system (primarily rest, digest, and recuperate functions).

Many breathing patterns are effective; the key is to use slow breaths, where the count for the exhale is no shorter than, and often longer than, the count for the inhale. We stimulate the sympathetic nervous system (primarily fight, flight, or freeze functions) on the inhale—resulting in a faster heart rate—and stimulate the parasympathetic nervous system on the exhale, which decreases how fast the heart beats.

When we're healthy, our breathing patterns produce steady and rhythmic heart rate fluctuations.

Having one or two breathing patterns memorized as calming tools is a great souvenir to take away from this Leg on managing stress.

Breathing Technique

Though the breathwork can be done pretty well anywhere, for maximum effectiveness, try to:

1. Sit in a comfortable spot, back straight (although standing or lying down, if comfortable for you, can also work with most types of breathwork).

2. Keep your tongue at the back of your top teeth.

3. Inhale through your nose. Exhale completely through your mouth around your tongue. If it helps, think of the exhale as blowing air out, with pursed lips, as through a straw, or blowing out a candle.

4. With inhalation, concentrate on expanding your abdomen vs. expanding your chest. Chest breathing can activate muscles in the neck and chest and trigger a sympathetic nervous system response. Belly or diaphragmatic breathing, using primarily the diaphragm, promotes slower, deeper breathing and can support a parasympathetic response.

5. I'll describe one breath cycle for each pattern listed below. Unless otherwise mentioned, repeat that cycle a minimum of three or four times.

Breath Exercise Options

Here are a couple of commonly used breathing patterns:

- Lengthen your exhale – This straightforward breath pattern option is to inhale as usual (don't take deep breaths or breathe too quickly) and then consciously spend a bit longer on your exhale. Try a 4-second inhale and a 6-second exhale. Expel all the air out of your lungs with each exhale, and then let the lungs fill up typically. This pattern can be done for 2-5 minutes.

- Box or square breathing – Start with a slow and complete exhale through your mouth to the count of 4. Hold there for the count of 4. Slowly inhale through your nose to the count of 4. Hold your breath for another slow count of 4. Exhale again, slowly and thoroughly, to the count of 4. Repeat the cycle, attempting to keep each count of 4 slow and equal.

- 4-7-8 – Developed by Dr. Andrew Weil, this technique acts as a, in his words, *"natural tranquilizer for the nervous system."* Close your mouth and inhale through your nose for a count of 4. Hold your breath for a count of 7. Exhale through your mouth, making a whoosh sound and completely discharging all air for a count of 8.

You can search online for additional patterns if you'd like to expand your breathwork repertoire. A few more options are alternate nostril breathing, abdomen or belly breathing, physiological sigh, resonant or coherent breathing, and yoga nidra (the latter falling under the more recently coined broader term, Non-Sleep Deep Rest or NSDR).

Chapter Twenty

LEG 6 - Metabolic Health For Life

SUMMARY - Travel Size Version

Where in This Leg, You'll Learn How to Finally Stop Talking Yourself Out of Doing the Things You Say Are Important!

*M*etabolic Health Roadmap is your chance to have your wellness efforts "stick." Anyone, for any number of reasons, can increase energy or improve sleep for a day, a week, or even a month. Following the Metabolic Health Roadmap system, however, with its simple, sensible, and sustainable approach to wellness, virtually guarantees metabolic health and vitality . . . for life!

And this is the Leg that solidifies the increased likelihood of that happening! We'll start with reminders of why wellness journeys so often abysmally fail and encourage you with why your chance of success—this time—is exponentially higher!

Diagnostic #5 - Set for Success Chart

The Set for Success Chart is your accountability-on-the-go tool. It's like a vacation fast food meal, but way better for you! Complete it for a baseline and then regularly (once/month) after that for simple, accurate feedback.

Where You Are

We'll review the Diagnostics in all 5 Legs to ensure you're clear on your *Metabolic Health Roadmap* starting point.

And Where You Are Going

Then we'll ensure you've got a clear idea of your destination—what you want to be, do (and later on, have and give). For ye of little faith (no shame there; I altogether counted myself in that category when I started my wellness journey!), you can even set your Faith Goals at a bare minimum level!

No Matter Whats

These are important! I'll give you a quick explanation. And I've listed three that are super important for everyone on the metabolic health journey. You might want to add a few more of your own.

Self-Regulation

We'll wrap up the book with a quick review of some of my own No Matter Whats, this time a significant condensing of what I consider to be important work in Dr. Bessel van der Kolk's book, *The Body Keeps the Score* and Dr. Joe Dispenza's book, *Becoming Supernatural*. If I leave you with nothing else, learning the value of self-regulation and the "how to" of self-regulation will be lifelong skills that will help you in every step of your journey.

Final Pre-Trip Checklist

Here's where I'll ensure you've got all the basics (passport, tickets, clean underwear!), and while you might be a little nervous and excited, you aren't feeling completely overwhelmed. I'll also give you some ways I can help support you after your metabolic health kick start!

Chapter Twenty-One

LEG 6 - Metabolic Health For Life: Getting Started

"Just because you can describe the gap doesn't mean you know what the problem is. You need to discover the obstacle that resides in the gap that is impeding your progress."

Keith J. Cunningham, The Road Less Stupid

One More Time. Why Do People Not Have the Metabolic Health They'd Like?

B y this point in the book, you will have some good ideas why!

First, they keep looking for new solutions to a problem that isn't there or, at the very least, the wrong problem. They can, as Keith Cunningham so eloquently states, "describe the gap." They are tired, brain-fogged, moody, discontent, and unfit.

And they gravitate to the "quick fix." They look for another diet. A new yoga class. A different gym membership. The latest mindfulness practice. But they've not gone deeper to discover the obstacles or, in *Metabolic Health Roadmap* language, the Road Blocks (wrong behavior) or Traffic Jams (wrong thinking) "that reside in the gap that is impeding" their progress.

So, mistake number two, without grasping the core reasons for the behaviors they exhibited in the past, such as:

- Abandoning their last diet and former gym

- Missing out on ½ of the classes in their previous yoga course

- Unable to be consistent with their earlier mindfulness practice

. . . they spend more resources—time, labor, and money—for yet more revolutions on the "trying to gain energy or fitness" hamster wheel rather than looking at root causes and enhancing overall metabolic health.

What Makes This Time Different for YOU?

Metabolic health only becomes possible with an understanding of the foundational reasons why a body hits the couch when it's walk time; a mind directs the making of a pot of ultra-processed mac and cheese when the fridge is stocked with veggies and grass-fed beef, and a spirit opts to binge the top-rated Netflix series the same day a new sacred explorations book, one was so excited about reading, arrives on the front step.

So, yes, understanding metabolic health is important, but even more, grasping how to grow in metabolic health ongoingly.

This Leg is about more than simply coming up with your next latest/greatest wellness game plan. It is about planning. It is about intentionally continuing to grow in understanding of who you are—genetically, body type, personality, and soul-wise. It is about discovering how the challenges in your life have fostered the protective mechanisms you have used in the past to stay as well as possible and how those mechanisms may no longer be serving you or keeping you well.

You Can't Be Responsible for What You Don't Know

And because of that lack of information, this Leg is also about making peace with yourself for the ways you've previously tried to be healthy. You didn't know what you didn't know. You did the best you could with the tools you had. But once you get new knowledge and realize there are new tools, it's choice time!

With the information you've learned in this book, you can now implement practices that foster the likelihood you'll do more of what you already do well. You also have the fantastic opportunity to do more of the things that allow your old and new brain to better cooperate in creating a shared vision and an actual "rubber meets the road" outworking of optimal health!

Lightbulb Moments are Important

I love it when my clients learn something new that they can use to optimize their wellness. I hope your list of revolutionary wellness steps to move you forward has lengthened considerably over the time you've read *Metabolic Health Roadmap*.

However, rather than feeling overwhelmed by that list of "newness," this Leg is about pairing existing wellness tools with small, manageable amounts of the new. That is a primary key to moving forward.

And Action is Where the Energy Is

So, while I'm a lifelong learner (and hope you are or become one as well), and the topic of wellness is a fascinating field with new research regularly being published, I didn't get where I am—from where I was—by reading and reviewing. I got here by what I put in my mouth. By how I moved my body. By the times I examined why I was behaving the way I was. By the times I was quiet and waited for "bigger picture" answers. By the times I turned off the light and went to bed earlier.

Less than optimal health is a symptom. The better you understand WHY you do things that contribute to that less-than-stellar health, the more likelihood you have of actually taking steps to improve it.

Diagnostic #5 – Set for Success Chart

This Leg's Diagnostic is a simple tool you can use (I suggest monthly) to check your progress with the Wellness Revolution Roadmap's primary and founda-tional BALANCE keys.

Complete the *Set for Success Chart* below so you have a baseline. By this time in the book, you should:

- Understand how you can better Eat for health and drink Clean water.

- Know your Body type.

- Have new ideas for incorporating more Activity into your life and have a rudimentary good Night's sleep routine in place.

- Be shifting in your Attitude (or at least understanding better some of the wrong information or thinking that influences your attitude) and adding more Laughter into your life so that you can work toward better self-regulation and stress management.

In the future, as you prioritize which Set for Success activity to habit hitch onto currently existing habits, please re-do the *Set for Success Chart*. It will help you evaluate areas still needing work and clearly show where you are reaching Action Goals. Those ongoing check-ups and slight course corrections are essential in reaching your optimal metabolic wellness destination!

SET FOR SUCCESS CHART

B-A-L-A-N-C-E	Action Goals Met			Not There Yet
BODY TYPE				
	Carb	Protein	Balanced	Don't Know
ATTITUDE				
		Think you can!		Think you can't!
LAUGHTER				
		5-10 Laughs/day		0-4 Laughs/day
ACTIVITY				
Fill in # of 15 min increments		Physical Activity		Non-work Screen
NIGHT'S SLEEP				
		Goal met		Goal not met
CLEAN WATER				
Fill in # of 8 oz cups		Goal met		Goal not met
WWR "Extras"				
Bowel movements		1-3/day		< 1/day
Hugs or "I love you"s given or received		1-5/day		< 1/day

Set for Success - Part 1

SET FOR SUCCESS CHART

B-A-L-A-N-C-E	Action Goals Met	Not There Yet
EAT FOR HEALTH	Balanced (optimal Fuel Mix, Comfortable Fullness)	Unbalanced (wrong Fuel Mix, too much or not enough food)
Breakfast		
Snack		
Lunch		
Snack		
Dinner		
Snack		
Sometimes Foods	1-2/week	> 2/week

CALCULATE SCORE

Add column 1 check two-page total and subtract column 2 check two-page total. Over time, work toward a higher score.

Column 1 Checks =   Column 2 Checks =

1_____ - 2_____ = Total _____

Set for Success - Part 2

Chapter Twenty-Two

LEG 6 - Where You Are; Where You Are Going

"Between stimulus and response there is a space. In that space is our power to choose our response. In our response lies our growth and our freedom."

Victor Frankl

INFORMATION CENTRE

A fter completing the book's five diagnostic tools (BALANCE Wellness Wheel, Dietary Needs Assessment, Snooze and Move Surveys, Paradigm SEE/SHIFT Priority, and Set for Success Chart), you should have a clear idea of your wellness journey's starting point.

Review them now so your levels, scores, and priorities regarding what to work on are fresh in your mind.

In this final Leg, we'll also examine where you are going, self-regulation as a tool to minimize pitfalls, and four final steps to optimal health per Bessel van der Kolk in *The Body Keeps the Score.*

The Destination

Now that you've gone through most of the book's Information Centres, I hope you have a much better idea of what your destination looks like in terms of what you will Be and Do when you arrive (and are already excited about what your destination can look like when you have time to discover Have and Give Faith Goals!).

Like when I started my journey, however, you maybe settled for a destination of bare minimums.

> *Can I please have less brain fog in mid-afternoon? Can I stop falling asleep on the couch the second I get home from work? Can I please be less irritated and snappy with the people I love? Can I be in a more comfortable-for-me body size without having to think about having food/not having food every minute of the day?*

When I started my journey, I could not have *conceived* of my current destination (or the one to which I'm headed next!).

Bare minimums are an OK place to start.

If you haven't already done so at Milestone #6 of your Roadmap, please fill in Be, Do, Have and Give as your Faith Goals categories. Then, have two (I'm suggesting Be and Do) fleshed out in your *Trip Log*. Feel free to dream big. If believing in big things is currently beyond your ability, then—like I initially did—set goals as the bare minimum of what you are hoping for.

But I'd also encourage you to create a second set of goals in your *Trip Log* beyond what you believe you can accomplish!

As best you can, design a set of Faith Goals that are bigger than you and that will require the support of mentors, coaches, friends who believe in you, and a source or higher power beyond you to complete. That's where the Faith part comes in.

Self-Regulation: The Gift That Keeps on Giving

Ultimately, the best gift you can give yourself (and those you care about) after a Metabolic Health Roadmap journey is to keep following through on your Seed

Habit Action Goals and understand how to regulate yourself and your emotions better.

Most Roadblocks and Traffic Jams have as their underlying "reason for being" a learned pattern of behavior caused by dis-regulation or incoherence in the body, mind, or spirit.

Excellent and helpful books, such as the ones mentioned in this Leg's Summary, are wonderful resources for a deep dive. Still, understanding that regulation requires work in both the emotional and rational brains is enough for a quick road trip.

Seed Habits Are Only as Good as Our Ability to Put Them into Practice

As mentioned throughout the book, how we come to self-exploration is extremely important. We've been making decisions and responding to events in a way that—based on our history and current situation—makes the most sense to us.

But what if that history and our brain's "stuckness" in that history creates helplessness and an inability to take action?

Like the rest of the body, the brain always tries to move toward increased health and homeostasis or balance. But, as previously discussed, that journey to metabolic health—energy, vitality, and optimal wellness—can be blocked. We can get stuck in powerlessness and become incapacitated.

Our emotional brain keeps secreting stress hormones. That puts the ability of the rational brain to give input and direction "on hold," as it were. Our emotional brain stays in charge. In essence, we are being directed to continuously defend against a threat—to our safety or to our best interests—that happened in the past and is already over.

Two Options for Better Managing Emotions

As Van der Kolk describes in *The Body Keeps the Score*, we need two critical types of work:

1. **Top Down Work** (responsibility of the rational brain)

   ○ Better monitoring of your body's sensations

2. **Bottom Up Work** (responsibility of the emotional brain)

   ○ Recalibration of the autonomic nervous system

HOW TO BETTER MANAGE EMOTIONS

Two important types of work are needed for healthy emotional self-regulation!

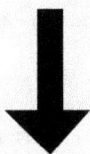

Top Down Work

The responsibility of the rational brain, top down work, entails better monitoring body sensations.

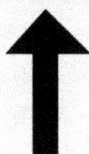

Bottom Up Work

The responsibility of the emotional brain, bottom up work, entails recalibrating the autonomic nervous system.

Per Dr. Bessel van der Kolk in *The Body Keeps the Score*

How to Better Manage Emotions

Top Down Work

Top-down work is simply asking your rational brain to pay better attention to the activity of your emotional brain. It can be easy for the rational brain to ignore the communication the emotional brain is sending. Top-down work—practices like mindfulness, meditation, and yoga—can help the rational brain more effectively monitor the many messages the emotional brain sends.

With that increased attunement, the rational brain can do the affirming (I hear you, thanks!) and calming (I'm on it and adjusting things!) work needed to keep the emotional brain from spinning in a sympathetic-dominant fight, flight, freeze, or fawn cycle.

Bottom Up Work

The emotional brain is where the bottom-up work needs to be done. Various types of breathing (check out the last Leg's Souvenir for reminders), movement (primal, dance), and touch (massage, tapping) are all helpful ways to switch from sympathetic dominance to a parasympathetic dominant response (rest, relax, and recuperate).

Realize, too, that the work is not either/or. Use a combination of tools that support both parts of the brain because while self-regulation is primarily the work of the rational brain, it is essential to strengthen the connection of that cognitive and executive function-focused part of our brain with our body. And with the body, it is primarily the emotional brain in charge!

Steps to Better Overall Health, AKA Van der Kolk's Steps to Change

The more I read about, study, and experience the ebbs and flows of physical vitality, the more I believe in emotional and spiritual growth contributing to increased metabolic health.

Yes, eating real food is an excellent place to start with metabolic health improvement (which is why we did it!). Still, long-term changes in our emotional and spiritual health will facilitate that energy's availability forever. Just like making dietary changes, helpful change steps can promote spiritual and emotional growth, too.

In *The Body Keeps the Score*, Van der Kolk lists four steps to change. I consider the change steps key to increased energy and optimal wellness so, as it is hard to describe the steps better than he does, I'll name them here and give an adapted description and version of tools to use to foster growth in each of the steps.

1) Finding a way to become calm.

- Breathwork

- Nature

- Music

- Dance

- Yoga

- Neurofeedback, EMDR (Eye Movement Desensitization and Reprocessing therapy)

Remember the last Leg's information about breathwork and its ability to take us from flight, fight, or freeze to rest, digest, and recuperate. Breathwork's stress management capabilities are why it is such an excellent calming tool.

Realize, as well, the many outstanding benefits of listening to or creating music, including the fact that singing releases endorphins into the brain. Dance significantly increases mental acuity regardless of how you do it (or look like while doing it!). And believe me, increased mental sharpness and awareness is a great way to help with calmness!

2) Learning to maintain calm and focus when triggered by past thoughts, emotions, and reminders.

- Mood-Thought Chart

- Mindfulness

- Relationships/support networks

- Prayer, chanting, practice of Namaste, meditation

- Focused visualization

Tools to help maintain calm and focus abound, including the classic behavioral modification Mood-Thought Chart, which can be helpful when emotions with deep ties to our past arise. I particularly like the original 7-Column Thought Record developed by Christine A. Padesky, PhD, in the late 1970s. I highly recommend getting a free copy/proper instructions on its use here: https://www.mindovermood.com/worksheets/).

Drawing on members of your support network, rhythmic prayer, and meditation have a long history of successful use. That use spans a wide range of geographic locations and faith practices.

Some examples include the Hindu practice of Namaste (Namaste is the practice of the divine—goodness—in me recognizing and honoring the divine—goodness—in you) and Gregorian chants (shown to lower blood pressure and reduce anxiety).

3) Finding a way to be fully alive in the present and engaged with others.

- Gratitude, looking for the good

- Top 10 List of Things That Bring Joy

- Knowing love languages

- Knowing body type or Enneagram

- Holding pain and goodness in tension

Gratitude and its signaling for the brain to release dopamine and serotonin—two critical neurotransmitters responsible for calm and focused emotions—not only helps with the second step to change but is also a well-used and studied tool for being more present and engaged.

Knowing yourself and others better (a joy list, understanding more about your own—and those close to you—personality and unique qualities) significantly impacts your ability to, in Dr. Joe Dispenza's words in *Becoming Supernatural*, be able to rest more fully in this "present generous moment."

The more engaged you are in your relationship with yourself, with others, and with your source or the divine, the more significantly enhanced your ability to change, including freeing up energy to give YOURSELF!

That depth of relationship also allows you to more easily (although, for me, "easily" in this regard is always relative!) hold in tension the areas where you differ in thought or opinion from others, as well as in the topics and decisions you are not yet quite, in and of yourself, sure about.

4) Not having to keep secrets from self, including how you managed to survive.

- Being objective in evaluating the tools you use to survive

- Being curious about how those tools came about

- Being compassionate with yourself

- Being gracious as you begin to make changes

And here we come full circle.

We are where we are primarily because of our self-protective and self-interest-motivated responses to things said and done to us or those we love and care about. Typically, those motivators have been hidden from others and often from ourselves.

EMOTIONAL STEPS TO METABOLIC HEALTH

Adapted from Bessel van der Kolk's Steps to Change in *The Body Keeps the Score*

1	2	3	4
Find a Way to Become Calm	**Stay Calm When Triggered by the Past**	**Be Fully Alive and Engaged in the Present**	**Don't Keep Secrets from Yourself**
Use breathwork, be in nature, play music, dance, practice yoga, use neurofeedback or EMDR.	Use a Mood-Thought Chart, mindfulness, support networks, prayer, meditation or focused visualization.	Practice gratitude, create a list of things that bring joy, know yourself, hold pain and goodness in tension.	Practice objectivity, curiosity and compassion about your secrets, including ways you have used them to survive.

Emotional Steps to Metabolic Health

One of the true joys of increased emotional, mental, and spiritual health is the way light can be shed on what has happened in our past and our reasons for our responses to that past.

It takes a LOT of energy to keep things in the dark! Light brings all manner of relief. The lifting of burdens. The breaking of shame. And then . . . the subsequent burst of energy and health that has now been freed up to use elsewhere!

Tell Me if it Works, if it Really, Really Works

I'm imagining my take on Spice Girls' lyrics is going to date me, but it would be worth it if I could really, really catch your attention right now!

It's crossroads time. You've done your diagnostics and assessed where your main wellness challenges lie. You've gained an overflowing tool kit's worth of simple steps to move you closer and closer to vitality and optimal wellness. You better understand why you behave and think the way you do, and you have the skills to both see and, should you decide, shift that behavior and thinking.

You now have to choose whether to leave the car in park or step on the gas and proceed with the necessary changes to ensure that your effort produces immense ongoing benefits and gets you to your destination!

Journal your decision to move forward. Reach out and tell a friend for accountability. Please email me at info@inbalancelm.com to pass along what you've decided (or for details on how I can best support you in your decision!).

Stories

I'm going to take a break from educating and, hopefully, instilling a little hope, and let a few clients—who decided to follow the metabolic health roadmap—take up the baton (I'd love to add your story to theirs!):

"Have felt more like myself than I have felt in the last . . . well, gosh . . . let's just say years."

"I used to wake up every 2 hours; now I sleep 5 or 6 hours at a stretch."

"Thanks for helping me get this brain and bod kicked into gear."

"I don't crave things like sweets and bread (instead, I crave vegetables!)."

"I have more energy, pride, and motivation."

"My energy is picking up . . . "

"I feel like the choices are getting easier."

"Your support over the years has made an incredible impact."

REST STOP

Time to take a break and digest information!

Take 10 minutes of calm to Rest with the following questions:

1. Do you likely need more Top Down Work or Bottom Up Work?

2. Which of Van der Kolk's Four Steps to Change resonated with you as an area needing further exploration?

Next, Stop for 10 minutes of quiet (sitting or slowly walking). Keep your mind as clear and open as possible, and just listen. Jot down any responses that may arise.

ROADWORK

Your next to last bit of RoadWork is pretty simple. Read the Traveller Assistance section below, grow in your knowledge of the concept of No Matter Whats, and then, per the directions you find there, begin to create your own collection of NMWs.

They stand the test of time (with little adjustments here and there), will become the framework for your Wellness Revolution Roadmap, and can easily be pulled out and dusted off should you take brief vacations from them.

TRAVELLER ASSISTANCE – No Matter Whats (NMWs)

"No Matter Whats" are Pretty Self-explanatory

They are the actions you take and the behaviors you respond to: No. Matter. What. And it's time to create a NMW list!

I imagine you'll want to start with a pretty small list because you may have a history of behaving or thinking that will make NMWs less than natural responses. I sure did! That's generally the whole point of carving them in stone!

Start With the Basics:

I suggest a couple of NMWs for each Leg and then prioritize that list so you can tackle just a few at once. Habit-hitch them onto actions you regularly do, and then, as those new actions become a habit, habit-hitch a few more.

For example, on the first page of your Wellness Revolution Roadmap, I suggested the following NMWs:

- An 80/20 ratio of Real to Sometimes Foods

- An increase in low-starch vegetables

- A minimum of .5-1 oz of water per lb/body weight per day

One or two of those are a great place to start for Leg 1, Eat for Metabolic Health.

Build on Those Basics

Once you have foundational NMWs in place and they are happening—No Matter What—then look to Leg 2 and add an additional NMW, body type-related. For example:

- Eat my recommended body type ratio of macronutrients 5/7 days a week

Once that habit has become a NMW, move on to Leg 3 Activity and Sleep NMW's. You get the picture.

NMWs Need Wiggle Room

Remember your Seed Habit keys—small, simple, sensible, and sustainable—as you create your NMWs. I also suggest ensuring your NMWs have "wiggle" room. That means having NMWs that have a range or are not required every single day of every single week for the rest of your life! NMWs with wiggle room look like walking at least 5000 steps five days/week, having four or five sugar-free days/week, and spending 10 minutes in mindfulness every other day.

We're not going for "perfection"; we're going for what produces benefit, what is manageable, what you enjoy (or eventually will enjoy, once you get used to it!), and what creates metabolic health. The Metabolic Wellness Roadmap is not a plan for simply gaining vim and vigor for the next six weeks or until you get tired of hearing my voice in your head, and try something new—this is Metabolic Health for Life!

Epilogue – Final Pre-Trip Checklist

"As long as we manage to stay calm, we can choose how we want to respond."

Bessel van der Kolk, M.D. The Body Keeps the Score

INFORMATION CENTRE

First, let me say that the "final," as in the Final Pre-Trip Checklist, is a fluid and ever-evolving "final!" Our emotional brain is not going anywhere (thank goodness). Your travel plans will need ongoing tweaking to facilitate growth in calming your old brain and creating additional ways for your newer, rational brain to pay attention when the emotional brain speaks.

But this Leg will be your final "official" session of the *Metabolic Health Roadmap* and the pre-trip steps you start with on your Roadmap to Wellness.

When All Else Fails, Check the Markers on the Roadmap

If you haven't already completed your Wellness Revolution Roadmap, *now's the time! It provides a great recap of your journey thus far and, in simple graphic form,* gives you a clear pathway forward.

Begin with road marker #1 and the chequered starting flags. At road marker #2, list the Eat for Health Leg's 3 Food Foundations and 5 Food Keys. Those will be your "coming home to real food" basics for whenever you get off track eating for your Body Type or have too many Sometimes Foods.

At road marker #3, list your Body Type and review the starting point Plate Portioning Guide graphic for your Body Type. You will want to continue to fine-tune your percentages to find the ratio of macronutrients that best suits you at any given point, but asking yourself how you are doing with:

- Physical energy

- Mental clarity

- Mood balance

- Bloating and comfortable-for-you body size

... will go a long way in helping you adjust to different stages of life and seasons of any given year.

Be sure your travel plans include road marker #3 No Matter Whats (for a reminder on those, check out the previous section's Traveler Assistance) and your most applicable Craving Calming Tip from Leg 2. Make liberal use of that tip's tools when cravings arise.

Next, be sure you've listed several steps of your new sleep hygiene routine under Road Marker #4. You'll also want to have made a note—in your *Trip Log*—of the Primal Moves you want to incorporate into your physical activity regularly.

At Road Marker #5, take note of whether you need more Bottom Up work or more Top Down work (calculating your Primary Stressors at that Road Marker will give you good clues), and then, at Road Marker #6, don't forget to complete your travel destination Faith Goals (including ensuring you've got a shortened Travel-Sized version with just the two Faith Goals you've prioritized).

Finally, get your habit hitching in place and remain open to continued question-asking, answer-seeking, and additional growth!

To Solo Journey or Not to Solo Journey? That is the Question!

Once your Wellness Roadmap is complete, the next task is to ask yourself if you are better off taking this journey on your own or better off getting a little guidance and support from someone who has "been there, done that!"

On the one hand, increasing energy and gaining wellness is elementary.

1. You sort through the reasons behind your present behavior.

2. Get your emotional and rational brains to communicate better with each other.

3. Come up with relevant Seed Habits for you/your body type.

4. Habit hitch those habits onto already existing actions you do well . . .

. . . and there you have it! Your epigenetic hacks to revitalize energy levels, sharpen cognitive function, cultivate emotional wellbeing and customize nutritional intake will foster increased metabolic health, and wellness "magically" starts to happen!

On the other hand, changing the thinking and behavior that produces energy and wellness can be challenging. The actions that must occur before the magic appears can sometimes feel daunting. You are:

1. Reducing exposure to cues that trigger the habits you want to weed out.

2. Increasing exposure to cues that trigger a habit you're trying to grow.

3. Trying new vegetables.

4. Aiming for more calmness.

5. Getting to bed earlier.

6. Being Objective, Curious and Compassionate!

And, sometimes, all that can be better accomplished with some help.

Therefore, I've provided a few extra online resources that you can review for additional support.

Bonus Online Resources on Tap

First, thank you for being here until the end! I don't take your expenditure of time and labor lightly.

And, as a sign of that appreciation (and also a way to pass along more encouraging words, concepts, and support . . . that didn't quite fit in this book!!) I'm giving you gifts!

First, access to 4 short videos that further unpack some of the most foundational aspects of the *Metabolic Health Roadmap*. You can access the videos through the links listed below.

1. Metabolic Typing Deep Dive

(https://www.inbalancelm.com/ESM_bonus-bodytype)

Twenty-five years ago, body typing or metabolic typing was brand-new information for me. When I started digging deeper into the topic, it was lightbulb-flashing, mind-blowingly life-changing! In this first bonus video, I'll expand on body typing and give you a few more critical clues to understanding body types' impact on digestion and sympathetic/parasympathetic dominance.

In other words, in the video, you'll get more specifics on how fueling for your body type benefits you both physically (Look, ma, no more afternoon slump!), emotionally (Who knew that wearing or not wearing my heart on my sleeve is tied to my body type?) and mentally (So I don't have to have a color-coordinated closet to be organized?).

2. Paradigms, Biases and Beliefs—Unwrapped

(https://www.inbalancelm.com/ESM_bonus-paradigms)

Because, in the *Metabolic Health Roadmap*, I've only been able to give you a "nutshell" version of how paradigms impact us—body, mind and spirit—in this video, we'll delve a little deeper into the topic.

I'll also explore a few more biases and underlying beliefs (because, trust me, it's super helpful to recognize any that are not serving you!) and give ways to SEE, SHIFT or MAKE PEACE with the additional paradigms as well!

3. Keys to Releasing Excess Body Fat

(https://www.inbalancelm.com/ESM_bonus-releaseexcessbodyfat)

You've read most of my thoughts on wellness throughout the book. Was it surprising that there was little mention of weight loss?

By now, I'm imagining you understand that it is because every body is different. We're wired for different heights, thicknesses and overall shapes. There is no "ideal" size, and trying to fit your body into a "one-size" societal-dictated mold is discouraging, sense-of-self-crushing and pretty much an exercise in futility.

There are times, however, that we carry excess and unneeded body fat—excess body fat we may choose to work to release. If that's you, this bonus video is for you.

In it, I'll explore the various reasons our body stores excess fat (not feeling safe, insufficient sleep, or, as some people do, and sadly queried by my younger self, "Eating too much ultra-processed food?") and some great keys to release it.

4. Holiday Hacks

(https://www.inbalancelm.com/ESM_bonus-holidayhacks)

Whether you are heading off on a two-week, all-inclusive vacation somewhere warm and sunny, getting ready to mark a birthday or anniversary milestone or prepping for whatever your family may celebrate in December, this bonus on Celebrating Well is for you.

We'll "hack" our way through the "holidays" with suggestions on how to keep the joy and meaning while minimizing the stress and anxiety and avoid falling into old patterns of protection, safety, and self-promotion!

Yes, you'll get a celebration clean-up tip or two (can you pair the word "celebration" with "clean up"?). Still, I promise to also give you lots of food for thought on how your holiday times and event markings can pull out all the stops with fun and goodness without leaving you with weeks of regret for the wellness ground you've lost. In other words? The best of both worlds: Celebrating Well!

BONUS VIDEO RESOURCES

1	2	3	4
Body Typing Deep Dive	**Paradigms, Biases and Beliefs**	**Releasing Excess Body Fat**	**Holiday Hacks**
Additional info on how optimally fueling benefits you physically and emotionally.	Discover a few more common paradigms and extra ways to SEE/SHIFT them.	Safe and wise ways to support your body to release excess stored body fat.	No matter the occasion, learning to celebrate well is key to optimal health.

Bonus Video Resources

Resources for Deeper and Accelerated Wellness Results

I only wish that when I started my "getting metabolically healthy" road trip, I'd have had the steps you've found here laid out for an increased energy and optimal wellness journey.

Simply implementing the plan and—with your newfound tools—dealing with the Roadblocks (wrong behaviours) and Traffic Jams (wrong thinking) that will arise as a natural course of living will deliver enhanced metabolic health and overall wellness.

However, if you want to go deeper on that journey or to have support in accelerating the wellness process, please get in touch with me through info@inbalancelm.com or my website at www.inbalancelm.com.

I love working one-on-one with the fantastic clients in my coaching practice. I also offer super helpful multi-week group coaching programs that support clients in moving toward physical, emotional, and spiritual transformation.

When that transformational process begins, I can support you in self-cultivating what you have learned so your body, mind, and spirit continue to flourish.

Head to www.inbalancelm.com and click the button requesting a free Wellness Roadmap call, or click HERE for direct access. I'll be in touch shortly, and we'll schedule a talk. Then, we can determine what might be the best fit moving forward.

Now it's time to move on to your last Rest Stop, RoadWork, Traveller Assistance and Souvenir. Thanks again for being here, and best of luck on the rest of the journey!

REST STOP

Time to take a break and digest information!

Take 10 minutes of calm to Rest with the following questions:

1. Who do you want to BE in five years? In five years, what do you want to be DO-ing?

2. What would you like to HAVE in five years? In five years, what do you want to be GIVE-ing?

Next, Stop for 10 minutes of quiet (sitting or slowly walking). Keep your mind as clear and open as possible, and just listen. Jot down any responses that may arise.

ROADWORK

Choose the option that most resonates with you. Note the option and your response in your *Trip Log*.

For many of us, dreaming has become a long-lost art. While, as children, we may have believed we could be or do or have or give anything, with—literally—no limits to our capabilities, over time and with a growing and more constricting set of paradigms, our dreams get smaller and the faith in our potential shrinks.

Time to Dream Again

Your RoadWork for this Leg is to become more expansive in your beliefs about your future.

Option 1 – Continue your Rest Stop work with additional "Dream" thinking and journaling, this time, explicitly asking yourself, "What would I love?" in the four categories of being, doing, having and giving. Consider your health and wellness. Look at love and relationships. Dream about vocation or passions. Examine your desires about resources (finances and time management). Then ask yourself these two questions:

- If resources (time, money or energy) were no object, "What would I love?"

- If I asked my 15-year-old self, "What would I love?" how would they answer?

- Look at the two sets of responses. How do they compare and contrast? What might need to shift?

Option 2 – Create a dream board—a visual representation of your Faith Goals and aspirations for life direction:

- List what you want to be, do, have and give in 3-5 years.

- Use text and visuals (pictures cut from magazines, photos, drawings you create, printouts of poems or sayings) to make a collage depicting what you'd like your future to look like.

- Post your dream board where you can easily see it each day.

Remember, Faith Goals, dreams, and visions are BIG. While with Action Goals, you mustn't be dependent on anyone else—or a time or priority-dictated request of your body—to reach your goal, with Faith Goals, it is OK if they require the uncertain cooperation of someone else or our body.

You can describe all the ways you would like to show up in the world, all the activities you'd like to be involved in, and the people—a partner, for example—with whom you'd like to be doing those activities. List the resources—time, energy, money—you'd like to have at your disposal and the ways you'd love to share them with others. All bets are off. Let your imagination run free and wild!

"To nurture our dreams and desires is one of the most important things we can do for ourselves. Our dreams are shaped by our desires,

*and our destiny is shaped from our dreams. . . . Often our long-held
dreams and goals or desires can fade to the background as our focus
gets caught up with day-to-day working and living."*

Unknown

TRAVELLER ASSISTANCE – Have a GROW Plan

. . . as in a Gutsy Recovery Of Wellness (GROW) Plan.

I help participants in my extended coaching programs create a GROW plan. It is a way to take charge of body, mind, and spirit wellness, even knowing—or perhaps more accurately, especially knowing—that there are always curve balls on a road trip.

Unbeknownst to your map and online app, the service station where you plan to refuel is permanently closed. Bridges get washed out. Mudslides happen. Accidents can occur, sometimes to you and sometimes to others, that disrupt the trip.

The curve balls can even be unexpected greatness! Maybe a wayside attraction calls your name, and the delay is actual, but the time loss is super beneficial in the long run.

Key to handling challenges well while continuing to gain insight into reasons for behaviours (SEE) so you can make healthier choices (SHIFT) is a helpful, dual-role, GROW plan:

1. **Reminder Guide.** A GROW plan acts as a second—less impacted by emotions—brain. In it, you list the Seed Habit Action Goals to which you're committed and the destination to which you are headed. A *Trip Log* or completed Road Map is an excellent first part of a GROW plan as it quickly reminds us why we started and why we continue moving toward increased energy and optimal health.

2. **Recovery Action Guide.** Due to the numerous undiscovered curve-balls already mentioned, you will get off track on your wellness journey. There will be weeks with packed schedules and holiday and seasonal distractions. You may sometimes feel self-doubt, overwhelm, or frustration at slow progress. A GROW Plan is your route to get back on the main highway to wellness. It's an IF/THEN guide that says, "**If** this happens, **then** I do this!"

What's the Plan to Get Back on Track?

With your Wellness Revolution Roadmap or *Trip Log* as a launch pad for your Gutsy Recovery Of Wellness Plan, all you need are the final touches of recovery action. Some suggestions?

1. **Plan immediate action** as the key to not letting doubting thoughts appear and nest in your hair. (If I have troubled sleep for more than three nights in a row, I'll review my bedtime routines and concentrate on taking additional sleep hygiene steps; if I have fewer than three sugar-free days in a week, I'll give myself a break from sugar for a week.)

2. **Have fun, uncomplicated methods** of tracking how you are doing (use the premade Success Chart, do a monthly colouring check-in on Leg 1's BALANCE Wellness Wheel or find an online app you like).

3. **Be gracious to yourself** both when creating your GROW Plan and when—as is normal and to be expected—you need to use it. Note my use of the word *when*. It's not a case of *whether* you'll ever need to enact your Gutsy Recovery Of Wellness Plan. You'll need it. Guaranteed. We all do.

A GROW Plan is a No Blame Plan

Since the only thing we don't know about getting off track is WHEN we will get off track, it makes no sense to allow our emotional or rational brain to play the Blame Game.

Therefore, we're not looking for a plan that points the finger at us for not keeping commitments, not being accountable enough, not having enough willpower, or feeling a sense of failure that leads to discouragement.

We want a GROW plan with an attitude of neutrality, normalcy, and acceptance of getting off track!

Please don't be lulled into self-judgement or condemnation. Take action to get back on track—and do that sooner rather than later!

Remember, perfection is not part of a wellness journey. We don't even know what wellness perfection looks like; witness the zillion—often conflicting in their information—health books on the shelves of your nearest big box bookstore! Success should, therefore, be measured by gradual progressive movement (and even include a few eye-opening setbacks along the way).

GROW PLAN

Put it into Practice:

1. Plan immediate action
   a. IF this happens/THEN I do this
2. Have fun, uncomplicated tracking methods
3. Be gracious to YOU!
4. We all need a GROW Plan

Gutsy Recovery Of Wellness

Grow Plan - Put it into Practice

One last thing before your souvenir gift ...

A Celebratory We Did It Review!

Wow, we've reached the end of our journey together through the "Metabolic Health Roadmap!" I hope you've found the tools and insights in this book helpful and that they've sparked some exciting changes in how you manage your wellness.

Now, I have a small favour to ask. If this book helped you see your health in a new light, please leave a review on Amazon. Your feedback not only helps me serve you better but also guides others who are searching for the same answers.

Leaving a review is easy:

Visit here: [https://geni.us/oR3NOXy] and share your thoughts!

Or scan the QR code below to leave your review:

MHR Review - QR
Code

That's it, except to say your support in this way is much appreciated! Now, on to your final souvenir!

SOUVENIR

Celebrating is a great idea when you reach the end of a journey, even a symbolic one like the one you've done in reading this book!

So, I suggest doing precisely that—celebrate—as your souvenir for this, the *Metabolic Health Roadmap*'s last (at least for now!) Leg! Dress up a little, maybe light a few candles, put on your favourite dance music and go for it! You might even want to prepare a few fun and tasty Sometimes Foods! And to help in the latter . . . enjoy my last gift to you.

Free <u>Celebration Foods Recipe Booklet</u>

Click the link or visit https://www.inbalancelm.com/WR_CelebrationFoo dsRecipeBooklet to download one of my favourite gifts to give to my clients, a collection of fun, meaningful, and tasty recipes to add delightful goodness to times of celebration.

Earlier, you got a taste preview of the recipe collection with my stepmom's Nibbles recipe. Now enjoy a whole bunch more sweet and—for those that don't do sugar—savoury Sometimes Foods options!

Until then . . . be well,
Brenda

About the Author

Brenda Wollenberg's extensive experience spanning decades as a social worker, co-leader of a faith community, and nutritionist is the foundation for her current focus on analyzing and interpreting body type and genetic data to create personalized wellness plans.

Brenda's expertise has been recognized on numerous platforms. She has been a guest on podcasts, her articles have been published in a diverse range of print media, and she has shared her knowledge in educational and corporate settings, showcasing her distinctive and compassionate approach to wellness.

As a decades-long partner to Mark, proud mama of five adult children, and nana to a growing gaggle of "grands," Brenda practices what she preaches with life-changing results!

References

1. Bailor, J. (2012). *The smarter science of slim: What the actual experts have proven about weight loss, dieting, & exercise.* Aavia Publishing.

2. Chandola, T., Brunner, E., & Marmot, M. (2006). Chronic stress at work and the metabolic syndrome: Prospective study. *BMJ*, 332(7540), 521-525. https://doi.org/10.1136/bmj.38693.435301.80

3. Clear, J. (2018). *Atomic habits: An easy & proven way to build good habits & break bad ones.* Avery.

4. Copinschi, G. (2005). Metabolic and endocrine effects of sleep deprivation. *Essential Psychopharmacology*, 6(6), 341-347.

5. Cunningham, K. J. (2018). *The road less stupid: Advice from the chairman of the board.* Austin, TX: Cunningham Group.

6. Dalton-Smith, S. (Speaker). (2020). *The real reason why we are tired and what to do about it* [Video]. TED Conferences. https://www.ted.com/talks/saundra_dalton_smith_the_real_reason_why_we_are_tired_and_what_to_do_about_it

7. Daubenmier, J., Lin, J., Blackburn, E., Hecht, F. M., Kristeller, J., Maninger, N., ... & Epel, E. (2011). Changes in stress, eating, and metabolic factors are related to changes in telomerase activity in a randomized mindfulness intervention pilot study. *Psychoneuroendocrinology*, 36(7), 917-928. https://doi.org/10.1016/j.psyneuen.2011.02.005

8. Dispenza, J. (2017). *Becoming supernatural: How common people are doing the uncommon.* Hay House, Inc.

9. Drager, L. F., Togeiro, S. M., Polotsky, V. Y., & Lorenzi-Filho, G. (2013). Obstructive sleep apnea: a cardiometabolic risk in obesity and the metabolic syndrome. *Journal of the American College of Cardiology*, 62(7), 569-576. https://doi.org/10.1016/j.jacc.2013.05.045

10. Feldman, J. *The Jay Feldman Podcast*. [Podcast]. Available at: Apple Podcasts, Google Podcasts, Stitcher and Spotify.

11. Gobry, P.-E. (2011, July 28). The 9 foods the U.S. government is paying you to eat. *The Atlantic*. https://www.theatlantic.com/business/archive/2011/07/the-9 -foods-the-us-government-is-paying-you-to-eat/241782/

12. Greenblatt, J. (n.d.). *Food addiction: Dairy and wheat*. Psychiatry Redefined. Retrieved from https://www.psychiatryredefined.org/food-add iction-dairy-and-wheat/

13. Hargreaves, M., & Spriet, L. L. (2020). Skeletal muscle energy metabolism during exercise. *Nature Metabolism*, 2, 817-828. https://doi.org/ 10.1038/s42255-020-00290-1

14. Hawley, J.A., & Lessard, S. J. (2008). Exercise training-induced improvements in insulin action. *Acta Physiologica*, 192(1), 127-135. https://doi.org/10.1111/j.1748-1716.2007.01783.x

15. HuffPost Life. (2011, July 27). Food knowledge is health power. HuffPost. Retrieved from https://www.huffpost.com/entry/food-knowledge-is-health_b_91067 6?utm_source=DailyBrief&utm_campaign=072711&utm_medium= email&utm_content=BlogEntry&utm_term=Daily+Brief

16. Irwin, M. R., Olmstead, R., & Carroll, J. E. (2016). Sleep disturbance, sleep duration, and inflammation: A systematic review and meta-analysis of cohort studies and experimental sleep deprivation. *Biological Psychiatry*, 80(1), 40-52. https://doi.org/10.1016/j.biopsych.2015.05.014

17. Kyrou, I., & Tsigos, C. (2007). Stress hormones: physiological stress and regulation of metabolism. *Current Opinion in Pharmacology*, 7(6), 607-617. https://doi.org/10.1016/j.coph.2007.10.010

18. Maté, G., & Maté, D. (2022). *The myth of normal: Trauma, illness, and healing in a toxic culture*. Knopf.

19. McLaren, B. (2021). *Why don't they get it? Overcoming bias in others (and yourself)*. Front Edge Publishing.

20. Miller, A. H., Maletic, V., & Raison, C. L. (2009). Inflammation and its discontents: the role of cytokines in the pathophysiology of major depression. *Biological Psychiatry*, 65(9), 732-741. https://doi.org/10.1016/j.biopsych.2008.11.029

21. Mind Over Mood. (n.d.). Worksheets. Retrieved [May 25, 2024], from https://www.mindovermood.com/worksheets/

22. Moss, M. (2014). *Salt sugar fat: How the food giants hooked us*. Random House Trade Paperbacks.

23. Mukherjee, S. (2016). *The gene: An intimate history*. Scribner.

24. Neff, K. (n.d.). Self-compassion. Self-Compassion by Kristin Neff. Retrieved July 25, 2024, from https://self-compassion.org/

25. Ørtenblad, N., Westerblad, H., & Nielsen, J. (2013). Muscle glycogen stores and fatigue. *The Journal of Physiology*, 591(18), 4405-4413. https://doi.org/10.1113/jphysiol.2013.251629

26. Ryan, A. S., & Nicklas, B. J. (2004). Reductions in plasma cytokine levels with weight loss improve insulin sensitivity in overweight and obese postmenopausal women. *Diabetes Care*, 27(7), 1699-1705. https://doi.org/10.2337/diacare.27.7.1699

27. Senate of Canada. (2016). *Proceedings of the Standing Senate Committee on Agriculture and Forestry*. Retrieved from https://publications.gc.ca/collections/collection_2016/sen/yc17-0/YC17-0-421-2-eng.pdf

28. Tzika, E., Dreker, T., & Imhof, A. (2018). Epigenetics and Metabolism in Health and Disease. *Frontiers in Genetics*, *9*. https://doi.org/10.3389/fgene.2018.00361

29. Ultra-processed food exposure and adverse health outcomes: Umbrella review of epidemiological meta-analyses. (2024). *BMJ, 384*. https://doi.org/10.1136/bmj-2023-077310

30. Van der Kolk, B. (2014). *The body keeps the score: Brain, mind, and body in the healing of trauma*. Viking.

31. Wolcott, W., & Fahey, T. (2000). *The metabolic typing diet: Customize your diet to: Free yourself from food cravings: Achieve your ideal weight; Enjoy high energy and robust health; Prevent and reverse disease.* Broadway Books.

32. YouTube. (n.d.). *Primal movement exercises* [Video playlist]. Retrieved [July 13, 2024], from https://www.youtube.com/playlist?list=PLsXV zsZHJJyBPIZCFOYY3cGdo9LJ_aL80

33. YouTube. (n.d.). *Stress Less Video Series | Physiological Sigh.* Retrieved [July 15, 2024], from https://www.youtube.com/watch?v=KxOSlR_ Mf-s.

34. YouTube. (n.d.). *Yoga Nidra and the Physiological Sigh | Nervous System Reset.* YouTube. Retrieved [July 15, 2024], from https://www.youtub e.com/watch?v=FYPPbMGkIW8

www.ingramcontent.com/pod-product-compliance
Lightning Source LLC
Chambersburg PA
CBHW062055270326
41931CB00013B/3079